HOW SHOULD I FEED MY CHILD?

From Pregnancy through Preschool

Sandra K. Nissenberg, M.S., R.D.

Margaret L. Bogle, Ph.D., R.D.

Edna P. Langholz, M.S., R.D.

Audrey C. Wright, M.S., R.D.

Library of Congress Cataloging-in-Publication Data:

Printed in the United States of America

10 9 8 7 6 5 4 3 2 1

DEDICATION

We dedicate this book to our coauthor Edna Page Langholz, who died shortly after completing her work on this project.

Without you this book would not have been possible. Your ongoing drive to try new ventures and make them fun along the way was the inspiration we needed to proceed. You were a terrific mentor, colleague, and friend and you'll be missed greatly.

Sandy Nissenberg

The vision, motivation, practicality, and sophistication were yours! The finished product is less than it would have been, but you were not one who looked back. We have benefited greatly from your friendship and know that the readers of this book will benefit from your wisdom!

Margaret Bogle

You were committed to excellence for yourself and those who surrounded you. Always generous with your time and talents, your vision for the future will be one of your greatest legacies. To reflect on the years that spanned our special friendship, I realize how fortunate I have been to have known and loved you.

Audrey Wright

Acknowledgments

The authors would like to thank Jane Tougas, Connie Holt, R.D., and the dietetic interns at St. Francis Hospital in Tulsa, Oklahoma for their contributions toward the completion of this book.

About the Authors

Sandra K. Nissenberg, M.S., R.D., is a nutrition consultant in Buffalo Grove, Illinois, and teaches classes and consults for the Buffalo Grove Park District. She is a former staff member of The American Dietetic Association and its Foundation.

Margaret L. Bogle, Ph.D., R.D., is on the faculty of the Department of Pediatrics, University of Arkansas for Medical Sciences, and Director of Clinical Nutrition and Research, Arkansas Children's Hospital in Little Rock. She has served on the Board of Directors of The American Dietetic Association and its Foundation.

Edna P. Langholz, M.S., R.D., was president of Langholz Consultants, Inc., in Tulsa, Oklahoma, and a past president of The American Dietetic Association and its Foundation.

Audrey C. Wright, M.S., R.D., is director of the Father Walter Memorial Center in Montgomery, Alabama. She has served on the Board of Directors of The American Dietetic Association and is past-president of its Foundation.

FOREWORD

How should I feed my child? This is the most common concern of new mothers and fathers even before the baby is born.

Today this question is even more important as we learn more about the impact of nutrients on a child—from a developing baby to infant to preschooler and beyond. Everywhere parents turn they are bombarded by scientific information about nutrition and children. One article says kids need this or that vitamin. Another report warns that some children are in danger if they lack certain nutrients.

But what does it all mean? The information is usually so scientific you need an interpreter. Parents need and want advice in commonsense, everyday words. They want to know how, what, when, and how much to feed their children. After all, parents want to provide their child with the best of everything—and that includes nutrition.

This book, *How Should I Feed My Child?*, translates the scientific facts into a commonsense approach to feeding young children. It is written by four registered dietitians who have worked many years with pediatricians, parents, and children. But best of all, the four authors are also mothers. They know all the nutrition facts in the world won't help you if Johnnie doesn't want to eat his vegetables.

The entire book is based on sound nutrition principles and scientific information, all geared to give parents specific, helpful tips. Starting with what nutrients are important for the mother during pregnancy, the book discusses the nutritional needs of the fetus, infant, and young child. Parents are offered specific examples of foods for their children and feeding plans. Of course, every parent will face some problems associated with feeding. The authors tell parents what to expect so they anticipate and prevent greater problems from developing.

The section on grocery shopping is most needed as we enter a new era of nutritional labeling of foods. More comprehensive nutrition information is being included on labels than ever before. Parents will learn the information they need to determine the nutritional quality of food. Plus, they're given insight into the advertising and marketing strategies of food companies.

This book also guides parents in establishing their role as parent—providing what food and when it is to be eaten—and allowing children to determine how much will be eaten. This concept, while getting much notice currently, is not new, but has been advocated by pediatricians for years.

The book's emphasis on breastfeeding and promotion of healthy eating habits for children and families is truly complementary to the nutritional advice that we as pediatricians attempt to convey.

I believe *How Should I Feed My Child?* will meet the needs of parents by providing sound, basic information in a way that can be understood and used. It certainly is a book I can and will recommend to my patients and pediatricians-in-training who can benefit from the authors' expertise and experience.

Betty A. Lowe, M.D.
Professor of Pediatrics, Dept. of Pediatrics /Associate
    Dean for Children's Affairs, University of Arkansas
    for Medical Sciences;
    Medical Director, Arkansas Children's Hospital;
    President, American Academy of Pediatrics

Contents

6. Smart Shopping 75

7. Eating Away From Home...................81

8. Fun with Food 87

Introduction

One of the greatest challenges we face as new parents is understanding how and what to feed our children. It sounds like an easy task, but it's not, of course. Children aren't just miniature adults who eat small adult meals. They have special nutritional needs. (They also have minds of their own and don't always know what's good for them!)

We all want our children to have the most rewarding and healthy lives they can. When they're young, that means we need to make good choices for them. And good nutrition is one of the most important areas in which we need to make thoughtful choices.

This book presents a commonsense approach to feeding your child beginning with pregnancy and progressing through the preschool years. Good food choices during the prenatal and early childhood years are important because they can ultimately lead to good nutrition throughout life. You'll learn to offer wise choices and select a variety of foods appropriate for your child. She'll then grow up with a clearer understanding of foods and how they're important to growth and health.

(Incidentally, you'll notice that we interchange 'he' and 'she' throughout the book. We think it's more appropriate than the traditional, exclusive use of 'he' and less cumbersome than using 'your child' or 'children'.)

This book covers your diet during pregnancy, infant feeding, introducing table foods, dealing with the independent toddler, preparing your preschooler to make good food choices for himself, food safety, special health concerns for youngsters, smart shopping, eating out, having fun learning about foods, and teaching appropriate table manners. We've also included a collection of recipes featuring new ideas and old favorites for your family. We conclude with parents' most commonly asked questions about feeding young children. Over 100 parents nationwide, including those with children in preschools, church groups, and day care centers, completed our survey on the subject.

This book addresses their questions and other nutrition concerns that most parents will face at some point. We are four registered dietitians, all mothers ourselves, with experience in nutrition and the feeding of young children. We have put the facts together for you in a commonsense approach, which we're sure will be a valuable resource as your child grows.

Happy, healthy eating for you and your family!

Sandra K. Nissenberg, M.S., R.D.
Margaret L. Bogle, Ph.D., R.D.
Edna P. Langholz, M.S., R.D.
Audrey C. Wright, M.S., R.D.

Chapter 1

Your Diet During Pregnancy

How will My Diet Affect My Baby?

You're pregnant! What joy! What an awesome responsibility. Yes, some things are out of your control—like whether your baby is a boy or girl, for instance. But you do have choices that could affect your baby for the rest of her life.

One of the most important decisions is your diet. You know the old saying, "You are what you eat." Well, as simplistic as it is, it's true. And for your unborn baby, that means, "She is what you eat." So unless you want her to be a cream-filled pastry, now's the time to make a commitment to healthy eating, if you haven't done so already.

It's best if you've had a well-balanced diet prior to your pregnancy and your nutritional status is good. Research has proven that mothers with good to excellent diets prior to and during their pregnancy have fewer complications during pregnancy, fewer premature births, and healthier babies.

In all three stages of pregnancy, the baby's development depends on the mother eating a well-balanced diet. In the first stage (the early weeks of pregnancy), the fertilized egg becomes implanted in the wall of the uterus. During the second stage, all major organs are formed. In the third stage, the fetus grows rapidly while the mother's reserves are established in preparation for labor.

You need to be concerned about more than just eating healthy foods, though. Your weight should be as close to the optimal as it can be at the start of the pregnancy. Being at your optimal weight allows you to concentrate on your pregnancy and corresponding weight gain without the added concerns of being overweight or underweight yourself. The following table shows desirable weight by height and size of frame, for women 25 to 59 years old, wearing 3 pounds of clothing and shoes with 1-inch heels.

Height	Small Frame	Medium Frame	Large Frame
4'10"	102-111	109-121	118-131
4'11"	103-113	111-123	120-134
5'0"	104-115	113-126	122-137
5'1"	106-118	115-129	125-140
5'2"	108-121	118-132	128-143
5'3"	111-124	121-135	131-147
5'4"	114-127	124-138	134-151
5'5"	117-130	127-141	137-155
5'6"	120-133	130-144	140-159
5'7"	123-136	133-147	143-163
5'8"	126-139	136-150	146-167
5'9"	129-142	139-153	149-170
5'10"	132-145	142-158	152-173
5'11"	135-148	145-159	155-176
6'0"	138-151	148-162	158-179

Courtesy of Metropolitan Life Insurance Company

What if you are over your optimal weight? If your pre-pregnancy weight is 20 percent or more above your normal range, you should reduce the number of calories in your diet. Some of the problems associated with being overweight include high blood pressure and diabetes. Another is carrying a large baby, thus complicating the delivery for both you and the baby.

If you are underweight at the beginning of your pregnancy (your desired weight is 10 percent or more below your optimal range), there are also special considerations for you. The possibility of an underweight infant and other complications could place you and your baby at risk.

How Much Weight Should I Gain?

Most of us resist gaining weight (at least we try to). But you can throw that idea out the window during pregnancy. You can expect to—and should—gain approximately 25 pounds if you are within your desired weight range as the pregnancy begins. This weight helps establish reserves in your body to ensure that the baby is at *his* optimal weight at delivery. It also lessens the possibility of complications.

If you are underweight, your doctor may suggest gaining up to 35 pounds. The best way to do this is by eating nutritious, high-calorie snacks between meals. Other ways to gain additional weight are listed below. If you are in doubt, a registered dietitian can help you establish a meal plan. And be sure to talk to your doctor if you have questions about how much to gain.

IF YOU ARE UNDERWEIGHT

- Eat regular meals with a minimum of three snacks.
- Use whole milk for drinking and in food preparation.
- Add non-fat dry milk powder to casseroles, soups, and prepared gravies.
- Use more margarine, peanut butter, and mayonnaise.
- Eat additional breads, cereals, potatoes, rice, pasta, and other starches.
- Choose nutritious high-calorie desserts, such as puddings, ice cream, milk shakes, and frozen yogurts.

Again, unless you are underweight or overweight, you should keep your weight gain to the recommended 25 pounds. Try to avoid fried foods, and limit butter, margarine, oils, salad dressings, and gravies. Unfortunately, the same goes for cookies, cakes, pies, and other sweets. To satisfy your "sweet tooth" eat fresh fruits and frozen or canned fruits without added sugar. More specific food choices are provided later in this chapter. Remember that exercise, as your doctor allows, will help burn excess calories.

In the first three months of pregnancy you should gain 2 to 4 pounds, which will come from consuming approximately 150 extra calories per day. However, during the second and third trimesters, a steady weight gain of approximately 1/2 to 1 pound *per week* is considered acceptable. To do this, you'll need approximately 350 extra calories per day. The weight gain from fat and nutrient storage is extremely necessary to meet the needs of good fetal growth in the last trimester, the demands of labor and delivery, and to prepare for breast feeding.

SUGGESTED RANGES OF WEIGHT GAIN

Weeks of Pregnancy	Weight Gain (pounds)
1 - 12	2 - 4
16	4 - 8
20	7 - 13
24	10 - 18
28	13 - 23
30	14 - 25
32	16 - 27
34	17 - 30
36	18 - 32
38	20 - 34
40	21 - 35

So where does all this extra weight during your pregnancy go? The following chart gives a little insight as to what is included in this weight gain.

PREGNANCY WEIGHT GAIN DISTRIBUTION

Tissue	Weight in Pounds (approximate)
Fetus (baby)	7 (may vary from 5-10)
Placenta	2
Amniotic Fluid	2
Uterus	2
Breasts	1
Blood Volume Increase	3
Body Fluid	3
Fat and Nutrient Storage	4
	22-27 pounds

What Foods Should I Eat?

Well-balanced meals and snacks are your tickets to gaining weight and getting the appropriate variety of nutrients in your diet. Your doctor will probably prescribe a prenatal supplement to ensure that you get all the vitamins and minerals you need, but this cannot replace a healthy diet from a variety of foods. Those nutrients that need to be increased during pregnancy include: protein, minerals (specifically calcium and iron), and vitamins that include B, C, E, and folic acid (folate).

Take a few moments to review the following food sources chart. Be sure to notice foods that appear more than once since they are rich in several nutrients. You might say they're the superstars of nutrition. With this information you can plan your meals to include foods in your diet that are not only good for you but also for your developing baby.

FOOD SOURCES & FUNCTIONS OF IMPORTANT NUTRIENTS

Nutrient	Food Source	Function
Protein	meat, fish, poultry, milk & dairy products, eggs, dried beans & peas	contains amino acids needed for building & maintaining body tissues
Carbohydrates	breads, cereals, pasta, rice, potatoes, sugar, honey, candy, fruit	major source of energy
Fat	oil, butter, margarine, meat fat, cream, nuts	provides energy, cushions & insulates body organs, maintains skin & body tissues
Fat Soluble Vitamins*		
Vitamin A	carrots, cantaloupe, greens, spinach, broccoli, apricots, pumpkin, sweet potatoes, milk, liver, eggs, butter, margarine	important for eyesight, essential for healthy skin, helps body resist infection
Vitamin D	fortified milk, egg yolks, cod liver oil (also sunlight)	important for strong bones & teeth
Vitamin E	vegetable oils, nuts, margarine, whole grains, wheat germ, spinach, cabbage, nuts	helps form normal red blood cells, muscle & other tissues; protects cells from damage

| Vitamin K | asparagus, broccoli, cabbage, lettuce, turnip greens, green peas | important for blood clotting |

* Fat soluble vitamins are stored in the body; excessive amounts taken can be toxic.

Water Soluble Vitamins**

Thiamin	pork, whole grain enriched breads & cereals, sunflower seeds, green peas, black beans, black-eyed peas, oatmeal, watermelon, winter squash, macaroni, peanuts	important for energy production
Riboflavin	milk, liver, meat, mushrooms, yogurt, broccoli	important for energy production
Niacin	milk, eggs, meat, poultry, fish, enriched breads & cereals, mushrooms, peaches, peanuts, potatoes	important for energy production
Vitamin B_6	meat, poultry, liver, pork, whole-grain breads & cereals, wheat germ	important in helping the body use proteins & fats
Vitamin B_{12}	meat, eggs, cheese, salmon, lamb, clams, scallops, wheat, nuts, lettuce	important for red blood cell development; functions of the nervous system

Folic Acid (folate)	spinach, asparagus, greens, lima beans, liver, black-eyed peas, pinto beans, navy beans, broccoli, beets	important for growth of tissues & muscles; helps in formation of hemoglobin (the iron-containing protein in red blood cells)
Vitamin C	oranges, grapefruit, lemons, limes, cantaloupe, straw-berries, melon, broccoli, green peas, brussel sprouts, spinach, cauliflower, tomatoes, cabbage, potatoes, sweet potatoes	helps fight infection; helps form collagen (the protein that forms the foundation of bones & teeth, scar tissues, tendons & ligaments)

** Water soluble vitamins are not stored long in the body. They are easily washed-out and must be consumed daily.

Minerals

Calcium	milk, cheese, yogurt, salmon, sardines, shrimp, spinach, broccoli, prunes, turnip greens	important for strong bones & teeth
Iron	meat, clams, eggs, oysters, liver, spinach, lima beans, peaches, navy beans, soybeans, kidney beans, asparagus, split peas, green peas	essential component in hemoglobin
Water	beverages, soups, solid foods	essential for transporting nutrients & waste; regulating body temperature

Most likely you won't have a problem getting enough protein because the American diet is usually high in protein. Still, pay attention to getting adequate protein during pregnancy because it is critical for growth.

Pregnancy makes your body scream out for minerals such as calcium and iron. These minerals enable the fetus to develop tissues and build bones. To boost your calcium intake, consume 3 to 4 cups of milk or milk products. To increase your iron intake, eat meat, enriched grain products, and dark green vegetables. Drinking vitamin C-rich juices (orange, grapefruit) will help, as well.

NUTRIENTS FOUND IN SELECTED FOOD GROUPS

Milk and Dairy Products

calcium, protein, riboflavin, vitamins A, D, and B_{12}

Meat and Protein Foods

protein, thiamin, riboflavin, niacin, iron, vitamins B_6, B_{12}

Fruits and Vegetables

vitamins A and C, folic acid, fiber

Breads and Cereals

thiamin, niacin, vitamin B_6, iron, fiber (from whole grains)

Probably the best overall guide to follow for a healthy, well-balanced diet is the U.S. Department of Agriculture's (USDA) Food Pyramid illustrated on page 115.

The USDA says approximately 55 percent of your calories should come from complex carbohydrates (fresh fruits and vegetables, whole-grain breads and cereals, and starches); 30 percent from fats (20 percent from polyunsaturated and monounsaturated sources found in vegetables, and 10 percent from saturated sources found in animals and palm and coconut oils); and the remaining 15 percent from protein (animal sources, such as meats, milk, eggs, cheese, and vegetable sources, such as legumes, dried beans, and peas).

In addition to the USDA recommendations, make an extra effort to drink more milk and eat more milk products. And skip the foods with no substantial nutritional value. Why eat the cotton candies of the food world if they won't help you or your growing baby?

What if Mom (and Baby) is a Vegetarian?

Many people today choose vegetarianism (eating foods primarily from plant sources) because they feel it represents a healthier lifestyle. However, a vegetarian diet can be challenging because it's harder to obtain necessary nutrients from plant sources than animal sources. Plus, there's added concerns if a pregnant woman consumes a vegetarian diet. She (and her baby) is at risk for deficiencies in protein, niacin, vitamin B_{12}, calcium, phosphorus, iron, and zinc. Still, with careful planning a vegetarian diet can include all the necessary nutrients.

The first consideration is to determine how restrictive your vegetarian diet is. Some vegetarian diets that include eggs and dairy products usually are not a problem. However, if your diet excludes *all* animal products, including fish, chicken, eggs, and milk (a vegan diet), you must carefully select foods to get the right nutrients.

You can get adequate protein from combining legumes (dried beans, such as black, lima, navy, pinto, kidney; soybeans, chick peas, split peas, lentils with grains), brown or wild rice, barley, soy or whole-wheat pasta, oats, and wheat germ at the same meal.

Brown rice, whole-wheat flour, dried beans, and peas will provide additional niacin. Calcium and phosphorus, usually provided by dairy foods, can come from tofu, soybean milk, corn tortillas, greens, and broccoli. Zinc is found in whole-grain cereals.

You may need to take iron supplements because the iron in plant sources (broccoli, spinach, greens, dried beans, and peas) is poorly absorbed by the body. Vitamin B_{12}, only found in animal sources, must be obtained with a vitamin supplement.

If you are following a vegetarian diet, be sure to talk with a registered dietitian who can help you plan appropriate meals to satisfy both your needs and those of your baby.

Common Concerns of Pregnancy

Morning Sickness

"*Morning* sickness?" many women ask. "Make that morning, noon, and night sickness!"

Yes, "morning sickness" is actually misnamed because nausea and vomiting can strike at any time of the day. And although morning sickness is very common during the second through fourth months of pregnancy, not every woman experiences it.

If you're not one of the lucky few, try to get up slowly in the morning and eat a few crackers or dry cereal. If nausea continues, we recommend eating high-carbohydrate, low-fat foods, such as dry toast or crackers with jelly.

Above all, don't go too long without food. Small frequent meals or snacks every 3 to 4 hours may help to alleviate morning sickness. Fasting, on the other hand, sometimes aggravates the condition. It also may help to drink your beverages between meals instead of with meals.

Certainly morning sickness is unpleasant and inconvenient. But it probably won't affect your health (and your baby's) if you are in excellent nutritional health and have ample stores of nutrients. As always, if you have any concerns about your pregnancy, talk with your doctor.

Leg Cramps, Fatigue, Heartburn, Constipation

Bouts of leg cramps, fatigue, heartburn, and constipation can be common during pregnancy. However, in many cases, the food you eat may help alleviate the problem.

The cause of leg cramps is not clearly understood, but they usually accompany fatigue or long periods of standing. Some women find that drinking more milk (which increases the intake of critical minerals) helps relieve leg cramps. Your doctor may even prescribe supplemental calcium as well.

If it seems like you're tired all the time, you're probably not imagining it. Fatigue is real during pregnancy and may cause decreased appetite, which causes even greater fatigue. Short rests, with feet up, lying down, are important. Plan ahead and increase rest periods during the day, especially if you are going to be up late. Adequate sleep (8 hours or more) is also essential.

Heartburn, which produces a burning sensation in the chest, may be caused by pressure of the enlarged uterus on the stomach. It may help to eat smaller and more frequent meals and less greasy and spicy foods.

The best relief for constipation is to eat more foods that are high in fiber and drink adequate fluids (6 to 8 glasses of water per day). Consuming 20 to 30 grams of fiber a day is considered a good intake. Foods containing fiber are noted in the following chart.

DIETARY FIBER CONTENT OF VARIOUS FOODS

Foods	Grams of Dietary Fiber
Breads	
bran muffin, 1 medium	3
whole-wheat bread, 1 slice	2
rye bread, 1 slice	1
Vegetables	
pinto beans, cooked, 1/2 cup	10
kidney beans, cooked, 1/2 cup	7
peas, cooked, 1/2 cup	4
potato, baked with skin	4
broccoli, cooked, 1/2 cup	3
corn, cooked, 1/2 cup	3
cabbage, raw, 1/2 cup	2
sweet potato, 1/2 medium	2
green beans, cooked, 1/2 cup	2
Cereals & Pasta	
barley, pearled, uncooked, 1/3 cup	9
bran cereal, 1 ounce	8
oatmeal plus fiber added, 1 ounce	6
spaghetti, whole wheat, 1 cup	4 1/2
bran flakes, 1 ounce	4
oat bran, 1 ounce	4
raisin bran, 1 ounce	4
oatmeal, 1 ounce	3
popcorn, 1 cup	2
spaghetti, 1 cup	2

Fruits & Nuts	Grams of Dietary Fiber
almonds, 1/4 cup	5
apple, 1 medium	3
banana, 1 medium	3
peach, 1 medium	3
peanuts, 1/4 cup	3
strawberries, 1 cup	3
cantaloupe, 1/2 small	2
orange, 1 medium	2
prunes, 1/3 cup	1 1/2
pineapple, 1/2 cup	1
raisins, 2 tablespoons	1

Special Cravings

The cravings of pregnant women have almost reached mythical proportions thanks to exaggerated portrayals on TV shows and in movies. Hollywood may not like it, but most women crave run-of-the-mill foods, such as milk shakes, ice cream, sweets, and pizza, which pose no nutritional threat or harm to the pregnancy.

Some women, however, crave non-food items. There's been reports that pregnant women have wanted to eat everything from ice and dirt to starch. If you crave any non-food items, you must seek your doctor's assistance. These types of items may cause digestion problems and thus nutrient deficiencies for your baby.

Don't hesitate to talk to your obstetrician about any cravings, morning sickness, or other pregnancy concerns you may be having. Early and routine prenatal care is vital for you and your baby.

Smoking, Alcohol, Drugs, Caffeine

Smoking is the most common environmental hazard during pregnancy. Not only can it affect the mother and baby during pregnancy and labor and delivery, but it can even affect conception. That means the best time to stop smoking (for both the mother and father) is before the pregnancy begins.

Primarily, babies of smokers are at risk of not growing adequately and thus having lower birth weights. Smoking interferes with the mother's blood supply (which carries nutrients to the developing fetus), so oxygen and nutrients are not carried to the baby as needed, thus causing retarded growth. Furthermore, if you smoke during pregnancy, your baby may have difficulty breathing, eating, maintaining proper body temperature, and resisting infection.

Expectant mothers should also avoid passive smoking (that supplied by other smokers). Being surrounded by smoke will increase your risk of ear, nose, and throat infections, bronchitis, pneumonia, asthma, and lung problems.

Alcohol falls into a close second behind smoking as an environmental hazard for pregnant women and their babies. Drinking alcohol during pregnancy adds greater risks of your baby developing fetal alcohol syndrome, an irreversible state of mental and physical damages, including reduced intelligence, hyperactivity, and eye and speech problems. Any alcohol you drink crosses through the placenta into the fetal bloodstream. Your baby's developing liver cannot metabolize the alcohol as your liver can, therefore the alcohol remains in his bloodstream long after it is eliminated from you.

Researchers are still studying exactly how much alcohol is harmful to a pregnancy, but the dangers of drinking alcohol are real. We recommend that pregnant women avoid alcohol altogether.

Drugs, whether prescription, over-the-counter, or illicit (marijuana, cocaine, etc.) also cross through the placenta to the developing fetus, just as alcohol does. Primarily, the fetus is at greatest risk during the early stages of pregnancy as its vital organs are developing. But drug use poses a risk at any stage of the pregnancy.

Pregnant women should discuss any prior or ongoing drug use with their doctor as soon as possible during (if not before) the pregnancy.

As for caffeine, there are questions about how much is safe. Pregnant women should limit their consumption of caffeine-containing foods and beverages (coffee, tea, cocoa, colas). Studies have shown that high amounts of caffeine can lead to abnormalities in small animals. Most doctors suggest eliminating or at least limiting consumption to once daily for the safest pregnancy.

Exercise During Pregnancy

So, you've made a commitment to eating a well-balanced diet and avoiding as many environmental hazards as possible, what else should you do during your pregnancy?

Unless your doctor restricts your physical activity, exercise should be an important consideration. Now, that doesn't mean you should take up a "new" sport. But you should continue the activity and exercise you participated in before pregnancy. You certainly do not have to lead a sedentary life for the next 9 months.

On the other hand, you don't need to "overdo" it with lots of exercise either. Put the Olympic training on hold, and especially avoid tennis, racquetball, or other jumping, bouncing, or excessively active sports during your last trimester. In no time you'll be getting plenty of exercise chasing after your baby.

Walking is by far the best exercise during pregnancy. There are exercise videotapes and classes for mothers-to-be that you may feel safe doing on a regular basis. As you enter the third trimester, your body changes will probably be the best guide as to what and how you can exercise. Be reasonable and sensible. Keep in mind that exercise and a nutritious diet will enhance your health and that of your baby.

Chapter 2

Feeding During the First Year

After a successful pregnancy and delivery of a healthy baby, you face some decisions about feeding your infant. What and how will you feed your baby? You obviously want to choose a method that allows physical, emotional, and intellectual development to proceed normally.

Your baby's first year is the most rapid growth period of her life. That's why it is so important to follow feeding practices that provide adequate nutrition and promote optimal growth and development.

Sometime prior to the birth of your baby, you should decide whether to breast feed or use commercial formulas (bottle feed). This is a family decision and should be discussed early. This decision is much too important to delay, especially since preparations should be made before your baby arrives.

Is Breast Feeding Right for Me?

Realizing that breast feeding is as normal as having a baby itself might be the first step in your decision-making process.

Human milk is a natural food for babies. Breast feeding can bring a sense of satisfaction to the mother and a safe, protected feeding to the infant. And research has shown that breast fed babies have fewer and less serious infections and illnesses. In many cases breast fed babies also have fewer feeding problems, allergies, and bouts of constipation.

There may be medical reasons why breast feeding would not be encouraged for you and your baby. However, these are unusual and few in number. Contrary to popular thinking, the size of the breast (small or large) and the shape of the nipple (inverted or small) does not prevent successful breast feeding.

If you have questions about your ability to breast feed, talk to your doctor.

ADVANTAGES OF BREAST FEEDING

- breast milk is adequate to meet the baby's nutritional needs.
- feeding allows a warm emotional relationship between mother and infant (bonding).
- antibodies and immune substances are present in breast milk.
- breast fed babies have fewer infections and illnesses.
- breast feeding provides less exposure of the baby to environmental contaminants.
- breast milk is convenient and always at the appropriate temperature.
- antibacterial agents are present in breast milk.
- no containers that require washing and sterilization are needed.
- breast fed babies overfeed less than babies fed formula.
- breast milk is more economical than formula.

Breast feeding is practical because it eliminates formula preparation and extra paraphernalia. You can always depend on breast milk to be the right temperature. And you can't beat the price, either!

Colostrum, or milk that comes from the breast in the first few days after birth, cannot be duplicated in a formula. This clear, yellowish secretion is not mature milk, but its unique characteristics give babies an immunity to certain infections during the first few months of life.

Breast feeding can be continued as long as desired. We recommend that babies be exclusively breast fed up to 4 to 6 months. If this is not possible, breast feeding for any length of time is recommended because of the mother-infant bonding and immune properties of the colostrum and early breast milk.

Breast feeding also offers important health benefits for the mother. Your infant's sucking causes your uterus to contract and return to normal size more quickly than when you are bottle feeding. In addition, the milk you produce comes from the fat stored during your pregnancy. Thus, breast feeding helps you return to your pre-pregnancy weight and shape while providing the best nutrition possible for your baby.

Because breast milk is deficient in vitamin D, you should check with your doctor to see if your baby needs a supplement during this time. A supplement may also be recommended if she is not exposed to sunlight (during the winter months, for instance).

I'm Not Sure How to Breast Feed

It's perfectly natural to be somewhat nervous to breast feed your baby at first. But don't worry. A little experience with techniques and positions will soon relax you.

Make yourself comfortable before you begin. Most mothers find it's more comfortable to sit—and hold their infant at a slight angle (head of infant higher than feet)—than lie down. Using pillows or sofa arm rests may help to bring your baby closer to your breast. Face his body toward yours for the best position for grasping your breast and maintaining eye contact. You can't help but look at that adorable baby of yours, eye to eye. Besides being one of the greatest joys of parenthood, this visual connection helps with bonding and builds a sense of security for your baby.

Babies are born with a reflex called rooting that causes them to turn their heads toward anything that touches their cheek or skin. Once you are in position, rub your nipple on his cheek that faces you and he will turn his face and open his mouth to grasp your nipple. Sucking begins as he has secured the nipple.

Babies suck pretty hard to obtain milk from the breast—at least harder than from a bottle nipple—so you may wonder whether he is getting enough. Usually 10 to 15 minutes on each breast will give sufficient milk. Be sure to allow your baby to suck from both breasts each feeding because this encourages a good supply of milk. Milk production is also enhanced with frequent feeding in the beginning (possibly every 2 hours) and when the baby empties the breast completely. Emptying the breast also benefits your baby because a greater concentration of fat in the breast milk comes with the end of the feeding (the hind milk).

It might help to make a simple chart to record which breast he began each feeding, since you should alternate breasts and begin with the other breast at the next feeding. (Placing a safety pin on your nursing bra strap is also a way to keep track.)

If your baby sleeps well and is active and happy, he's probably receiving an adequate amount of breast milk.

Most hospitals have professionals (sometimes referred to as "lactation consultants") that will teach you the techniques of breast feeding before you are discharged. They can also give you a number to call with questions after you are home with your infant. Don't hesitate to ask for help or suggestions.

Help is also available in most cities from the La Leche League, an organization of nursing mothers whose purpose is to support breast feeding worldwide. La Leche League usually offers classes for the expectant mother and can help nursing mothers if they encounter a problem at home. Other breast feeding mothers can offer support and give suggestions on practical aspects of feeding, pumping, and scheduling.

What About When I'm Away?

It's going to happen. As much as you adore your little one, you'll need be away from her. Perhaps you're returning to work or maybe you just need an afternoon for yourself. Whatever the case, there should not be long periods without sucking (or pumping). The continued production of milk works on a supply and demand system—so the less she gets, the less you produce, and vice versa.

Pumping the breasts will provide milk for her when you are away for several hours and a sitter or dad is handling the feeding duties. Breast fed babies will usually accept a bottle when they discover it has the familiar breast milk in it.

Fortunately, as the popularity of breast feeding increases, more and more employers are providing space and time for mothers to breast feed or pump their breasts for later feedings. Breast feeding on the job or pumping the breasts will ensure an adequate amount of mother's milk.

Information on appropriate pumps and techniques for using them is available from lactation consultants, La Leche League, individuals renting pumps, or pump manufacturers. Check the telephone book or call your local hospital for information.

The following tips may help you with any additional breast feeding concerns:

- The majority of mothers can produce enough milk.
- Twins and triplets can be successfully breast fed if scheduled properly.
- Starting to breast feed immediately after birth stimulates the production of breast milk. Putting baby to the breast for sucking at regular intervals will increase the production and supply of milk. The supply of milk comes in direct proportion to the sucking efforts of the infant.
- Frequent sucking helps to stop the breasts from becoming swollen and painful. This relieves engorgement.
- The size of the breast does not make a difference in breast feeding or volume of milk. Mothers with small breasts can produce adequate amounts of milk.
- Breast milk meets the nutritional needs of healthy newborns. The nutrient quality of breast milk continues to be adequate during the first 4 to 6 months.

- Continuing the good eating habits of pregnancy will provide good nutrition for breast feeding.
- Breast feeding fosters a close emotional bond between mother and child.
- Breast feeding usually helps the mother regain her figure more quickly.
- Breast feeding does not make breasts sag.
- Medications should be checked by a doctor because some are transferred into breast milk and could be harmful to your baby.
- Breast feeding can be continued as long as desired but it is recommended to last at least 4 to 6 months.
- Caffeine-containing beverages should be limited and alcohol avoided.
- For the volume of breast milk to be adequate, the mother should drink plenty of liquids, including water, milk, and fruit juices.

Sometimes My Baby Seems Fussy When She Nurses

Remember our discussion on the old saying, "You are what you eat"? Well, it also applies to breast milk. If your baby becomes fussy while eating she may be reacting to the milk. Flavors of food you eat will be passed to your baby through the breast milk.

Spicy foods, onions, and garlic particularly will change the flavor of breast milk and are not always enjoyed by babies. You'll be the judge of what works and which should be eliminated, although it may take a lot of trial and error.

Still, some mothers notice no reactions in their babies and continue to eat whatever they want. As you already know from talking to other parents, each baby is an individual and some will tolerate what others will not.

Other substances, such as drugs of abuse, medications, caffeine, and alcohol, may appear in mother's milk. In particular, alcohol and caffeine appear in breast milk at the same levels as in the mother's bloodstream. They should be consumed in moderation and avoided immediately before breast feeding. Your doctor can tell you more about which drugs to avoid during breast feeding.

What About Commercial Formulas?

No mother should feel inferior or inadequate if she chooses not to breast feed her infant. Numerous formulas are available to substitute for breast milk. These formulas provide for adequate growth, and bonding occurs easily with bottle feedings.

All commercial formulas are similar in nutrient content. However, you should choose an iron fortified formula because your baby will need more iron in the first 4 to 6 months than he can get from milk alone. Formula comes in three types—ready-to-feed, liquid concentrate, or dry powdered. Many mothers prefer ready-to-feed commercial formula because it is easy to use and requires no mixing or additives; just pour it from the can and serve. Of course, you'll pay more for the convenience.

Most formulas are made from modified cow's milk. If you or your family has a history of allergies to cow's milk, talk to your doctor before choosing a formula. There are iron fortified formulas made from soy protein that can be substituted for regular formulas, but your doctor should make that decision. Your baby's formula should not be changed without your doctor's knowledge because frequent changes could upset your baby and his appetite. (More information about changing formulas appears on page 26.) Talk to your doctor immediately if you question your baby's tolerance of his formula (he has diarrhea, gas, vomits, etc.).

There are other therapeutic formulas (protein hydrolysate, elemental, and modular) available for specific diseases or medical conditions. Although these are available from retail pharmacies, they must not be used without your doctor's prescription and monitoring. It is beyond the scope of this book to detail the specific uses of therapeutic formulas.

There are a variety of baby bottles on the market: glass, plastic, and plastic with disposable bags. They come in all colors, shapes, and sizes. Most common sizes are 4 ounces (to be used when baby is taking less than 4 ounces per feeding) and 8 ounces (to be used as baby drinks more at each feeding). Do not get hung up on what kind of bottle to use. They all work equally well. One advantage of plastic is that it is lightweight and unbreakable—something to think about when your baby is trying to hold her own bottle, over your kitchen floor.

The upper rack of the dishwasher is excellent for cleaning bottles and nipples. Rinse the bottles and nipples with cold water before putting them into the dishwasher. Nipples and bottle covers and caps should be placed in a small covered plastic basket before putting them into the dishwasher.

Babies have limited protection against infection, so take special care in formula preparation and feeding. Formula is an excellent medium for bacteria, which could cause diarrhea or other problems. Use extra sanitary precautions: clean hands and utensils, refrigerate formula after preparation, and throw out any formula that has been left at room temperature for 2 hours.

Although it's more convenient to mix a 24-hour supply of bottles at one time and store them in the refrigerator, some mothers prefer to mix one bottle at a time. This way the formula is near room temperature and requires no heating. Actually, babies do not care if the formula is cold and it is digested equally well cold or warm.

Remember, once you have warmed a bottle of formula (or if it is at room temperature) and fed your baby, any unused formula should be thrown away. Do not try to get her to finish every drop—this is one time when baby knows best. The most common cause of overfeeding is mom trying to get baby to completely empty every bottle. If your baby stops drinking before the bottle is empty, it simply means you overestimated how much she would take at that feeding.

FORMULA FEEDING TIPS

- Wash outside of formula can. Be sure your hands and all dishes used are clean.

- Sterilize bottles in boiling water or in a dishwasher.

- Mix formula with water according to directions on can. Only ready-to-feed formula requires no additional water.

- Fill bottles to desired level; enough for one feeding.

- Cover nipples to keep clean.

- Place bottles in refrigerator until ready to use. Use bottles within a 24-hour period.

- Formula can be fed cold or warmed (baby does not care).

- If warming a bottle, use an electric warmer, or heat water in the microwave, placing bottle in the hot water after removing the water from the microwave.

- Do not warm bottles in microwave ovens. Bottles will develop hot spots. Formula is hotter than you think, and baby can get burned from overheated milk.

- Do not return unused formula to the refrigerator after warming. Bacteria grows at room temperature and higher. Your baby could become sick from reused formula.

- Bottles are easier to clean if rinsed immediately after use.

- For ease in feeding, keep a 24-hour supply of formula in the refrigerator.

- If traveling for several hours, keep bottles of formula in an ice chest to keep them cool and prevent bacterial growth.

Always hold your baby for bottle feedings. And let dad take his turn, too. Babies need this closeness for psychological, safety, and security reasons. Propped bottles can over feed or cause a baby to choke. The bottle should be held in such a way that liquid fills the end of the nipple with no air space, otherwise your baby will swallow air that can cause "spit up" or "colic."

In the first month, your baby will probably take six to ten small bottles a day of formula (2 to 3 ounces each). You should burp him (bring up air) after each ounce or ounce and a half of formula. As he gets older, he'll gradually drink more and more per bottle and not have to feed so frequently. The time between "burps" can also be lengthened to 2 ounces, 4 ounces, 6 ounces, and finally, after each 8-ounce bottle. Burping can be done by laying him face down on your shoulder and gently rubbing or patting his back. You can also hold him upright (supporting the head) on your lap and gently rub his back until the air is brought up.

Can I Change Formulas?

Once you and your doctor have selected an iron fortified formula for your baby, relatives, other mothers, and friends—even the grocery store clerk—may suggest changing formulas for one reason or another. Do not change formulas without consulting your doctor. Remember, well-meaning friends and their babies are different from yours.

Some may tell you that iron fortified formulas cause problems with digestion, increased gas, diarrhea, or constipation. These are myths. Numerous well-controlled studies have proven that the only difference between iron fortified formula and other formula is the color of the bowel movement produced. Bowel movements of babies on iron fortified formula will be darker in color. Just be sure the formula is diluted correctly with water since lack of adequate water may contribute to constipation.

When Can I Offer Milk?

Wait until your baby is at least one before serving her unmodified cow's milk (homogenized whole). As she begins to have good trunk control and sits alone, give her breast milk or formula in a non-breakable cup or small glass to prepare for weaning. A tippy cup is OK in the beginning to avoid spills but it still requires the sucking skill. By 6 months, she should accept liquids from an open glass. If she uses a tippy cup too long, it becomes a habit that may take 2 or 3 years to break.

Even if your baby is weaned from the bottle during the last 2 to 3 months of the first year, continue serving formula from a non-breakable cup or small glass. Whole milk can be offered to 1- to 2-year-old children. Two percent or skim milk is not recommended until after the second birthday because it does not provide enough energy and is much more difficult to digest for infants.

What About Water?

Water is an important nutrient that carries nutrients to cells and waste products out of the body. It aids in digestion and metabolism, and regulates body temperature. However, because formulas contain a lot of water, your baby doesn't need extra water unless the weather is warm (summertime). *Plain* water should be offered once or twice per day during hot weather. We emphasize *plain* because parents sometimes add sugar, syrup, or honey to their child's water. This is a mistake, though, because he'll want the sweet taste all the time.

When Do I Begin Baby Foods?

Breast milk and iron fortified formula provide all the nutrients your baby needs for the first 4 to 6 months when his digestive system is not ready for any food other than milk. But before you know it, your tiny one will be ready for solid foods. At about 4 to 6 months he'll start to have good control of his head, neck, and upper body. You'll know he's ready for strained baby foods when he can control his head while sitting and transfer solids from the front of his mouth to the back and swallow.

At first his normal tongue thrust will push foods from the mouth. Don't worry, though, it's not that he doesn't like the taste of the food—he's just resisting new textures in his mouth. Accepting and moving solid foods to the back of the mouth for swallowing is tricky. It's part learned behavior and part developmental skills. Differences in textures, thick or runny, are not accepted quickly. He'll get used to different textures over time, just keep trying new foods. It's not until much later in the first year that babies start making choices based on tastes other than sweetness.

It's best to start with rice cereal, which is easily digested, iron fortified, and hypoallergenic. Mix the cereal with formula until it is slightly thicker than formula (consistency of applesauce) and feed your baby in tablespoon increments. All baby foods should be fed with a spoon. Never serve baby foods from a bottle or syringe-type feeder. After two weeks on rice cereal, try serving oatmeal or other plain cereal. Mixed cereals should not be served until at least two plain cereals are tolerated. Cereals and other foods should be offered one at a time over 2 to 3 days. This way, you'll know if he tolerates that food. And if there are problems, you'll be able to identify which food is causing the problem and eliminate it.

After two or more cereals have been fed, vegetables may be offered. Each new food should be offered in small amounts two to three times daily, using the same food for at least 3 days before trying another food. A guide for introducing solid foods follows, and more information on weaning appears on page 36.

INTRODUCING SOLID FOODS

Age	Foods
4 to 5 months	iron fortified cereals (rice, oatmeal, mixed)
5 to 6 months	strained vegetables (yellow and green)
6 to 7 months	strained fruits and juices (peaches, applesauce, pears)
7 to 8 months	strained meats (chicken, turkey, beef, pork)
8 to 9 months	strained or mashed hard cooked egg yolk

All along we've talked about how important your child's diet is for her development. Here's a perfect example; children who are offered cereal and vegetables before fruits (which are sweeter) are more likely to eat more vegetables than children who get fruits before vegetables.

At this age, babies prefer plain cereals and single vegetables and fruits over mixtures. Plus, if he doesn't tolerate some foods, it is more quickly identified if only plain foods are offered. Don't be concerned about needing to offer a large variety of cereals, vegetables, or fruits. You'll become bored with carrots or rice cereal long before your baby does. Babies' taste buds are just developing and are not used to the variety you have experienced. More variety in foods can come after you're sure he's tolerating individual foods.

Fruit juices (2 to 4 ounces at a time daily), diluted with water at first, can be added as fruits are offered. But don't allow fruit juice to replace breast milk or formula. Use juices that do not have sugar added. Some of the dark fruits like strained prunes and plums seem to be useful in preventing or treating constipation.

SUGGESTED DAILY FEEDING SCHEDULE

TIME	4-5 months	5-6 months	6-7 months	8-9 months	10-12 months
Early Morning (waking)	4 oz. formula*	4 oz. formula	4 oz. formula	4 oz. formula or juice	4 oz. formula or juice
8-9 a.m.	1-2 T. dry cereal mixed with formula Wk I rice Wk II oatmeal Wk III mixed Wk IV rice 2-3 oz. formula	1-2 T. dry cereal** 2-3 oz. formula	3-4 T. dry cereal** Wk I (1-2 T.) applesauce Wk II peaches Wk III pears Wk IV bananas 2-3 oz. formula	3-4 T. dry cereal** 2-3 T. fruit 2-3 oz. formula	4-5 T. dry cereal** 1 jar fruit 1-2 T. egg yolk 2-3 oz. formula
Mid-Day	1-2 T. dry cereal mixed with formula Wk I rice Wk II oatmeal Wk III mixed Wk IV rice 2-3 oz. formula	1-2 T. vegetables Wk I carrots Wk II green beans Wk III peas Wk IV squash 3-4 oz. formula from a cup or glass	2-3 T. vegetables 1-2 T. fruit Wk I applesauce Wk II peaches Wk III pears Wk IV bananas 3-4 oz. formula from a cup or glass	1/2 to 1 jar vegetables 1/2 to 1 jar fruit 1-2 T. meat Wk I chicken Wk II turkey Wk III beef Wk IV liver 3-4 oz. formula from a cup or glass	1/2 to 1 jar vegetables 1/2 to 1 jar fruit 1/2 jar meat 4-6 oz. formula from a cup or glass

TIME	4-5 months	5-6 months	6-7 months	8-9 months	10-12 months
Mid-Afternoon	6 oz. formula	2-4 oz. formula or veg. juice Wk I carrot juice Wk II mixed veg. juice	2-4 oz. formula or fruit juice Wk I apple juice Wk II orange juice Wk III pear juice Wk IV mixed juice	2-4 oz. juice 4-6 oz. formula	2-4 oz. juice 4-6 oz. formula
Dinner	1-2 T. dry cereal mixed with formula Wk I rice Wk II oatmeal Wk III mixed Wk VI rice 2-3 oz. formula	1-2 T. dry cereal** 1-2 T. vegetables Wk I carrots Wk II green beans Wk III peas Wk IV squash 3-4 oz. formula	1-2 T. dry cereal** 2-3 T. vegetables 1-2 T. fruit Wk I applesauce Wk II peaches Wk III pears Wk IV bananas 3-4 oz. formula	1/2 to 1 jar vegetables 1/2 to 1 jar fruit 1-2 T. meat Wk I chicken Wk II turkey Wk III beef Wk IV liver 3-4 oz. formula	1/2 to 1 jar vegetables 1/2 to 1 jar fruit 1/2 to 1 jar meat or egg yolks 3-4 oz. formula
Bedtime	6 oz. formula	6 oz. formula	6 oz. formula	6 oz. formula	6 oz. formula

* Breast milk can be substituted for formula.

** Mixed with formula or breast milk.

Strained meats are good sources of iron. Strained meats and cooked egg yolk are introduced last primarily because of their texture, which is thicker than strained fruits and vegetables and less smooth—not exactly a favorite combination for babies. You may want to thin meats and cooked egg yolks with a small amount of formula to make them more acceptable to your baby.

Strained foods can be fed at room temperature or slightly warmed. If foods are warmed, throw out the leftovers after each feeding. You should spoon the foods onto a saucer or small bowl before feeding. If you feed from the jar, your baby's saliva on the spoon will mix with the food in the jar and make it thin and watery. (Enzymes in saliva begin digesting food whether the food is in her mouth or in the jar.)

As strained foods are being introduced, it's important to read labels and buy or prepare single ingredient foods (rice cereal, green beans, applesauce, chicken). With mixtures (vegetable dinners, high meat dinners, puddings), it's difficult to determine the nutrient value and your baby can't distinguish between flavors. Also, as we discussed earlier, single ingredient foods allow you to pinpoint any tolerance problems. Later, after all types of foods are being eaten, you can offer mixtures of foods.

Commercially prepared strained foods are convenient, contain few, if any, additives, and are good sources of all nutrients. Read labels and skip the foods that have added salt or sugar. Your baby doesn't need it. It's also a good idea to resist the temptation to taste the strained foods. Believe us, they'll taste extremely bland to your adult taste buds and you may want to add margarine, salt, or sugar, which your infant does not need.

Making Homemade Strained Food

You may want to puree foods for your baby when you introduce solids (at 4 to 6 months). Fresh and frozen fruits and vegetables can be steamed or stewed without added salt, margarine, or butter.

If you're cooking for the family, set aside a small portion of the vegetable for your baby before seasoning is added. (Leftovers from the family table are usually too highly seasoned.) Puree the food for your baby in a blender and freeze the surplus for later use. Remember that babies need to distinguish flavors so puree fruits and vegetables individually. Pour the puree into ice cube trays or plastic bags for freezing. These make ideal portions and once frozen can be stored, labeled, and dated. Just take out the number of frozen cubes you need at each feeding.

Pureeing your own foods begins with vegetables because they're the next food offered after strained cereals. Vegetables can be cooked in homemade chicken broth or plain water until tender and then pureed, adding a small amount of the broth, if necessary, back into the mixture while blending. Carrots, potatoes, squash, green beans, spinach, and peas usually work best.

Fresh fruits or canned fruits (either packed in their own juice or water packed) also make good purees. Most babies like pears, applesauce, peaches, and bananas the most. As mentioned before, avoid using fruits canned in sugar syrups.

When your little tyke has progressed to eating meat, try stewing the meat in water to first make a broth that can be used as a liquid in pureeing. However, do not add salt.

A point to remember about meat, especially beef, chicken, or pork, is that it has many fibers that can make it difficult to achieve a fine puree. You may have to cut the meat into small pieces or even coarsely grind it before stewing. This not only reduces its stringy consistency, but also allows for better softening in the cooking process.

Finger Feeding

Your baby's whirlwind first year is coming to an end now as she's getting better at sitting (using a high chair) and moving her hands to her mouth. This is the time (around 9 to 12 months) when you should offer your baby appropriate finger foods that may require some chewing motions. Pieces of soft-cooked vegetables or canned fruits, zwieback, or oven-dried toast are good first finger foods. At this age your baby can also hold a small glass with both hands and drink small amounts by herself—and get her cheeks wet. (A quick tip: a small amount in the glass makes for less mess if spilled.)

Let your baby try to use a short-handled spoon that she can grasp in a fist. But make sure there's something thick on the plate she can dig the spoon into (mashed potatoes, thickened cereal). Liquids or runny foods will be spilled because she will naturally turn the spoon over on the way to the mouth until after she is 1 year of age.

Until your baby is skilled at feeding herself and using a spoon, you can expect some playing in the food and messiness. (Use large terry cloth bibs to cover clothing. These can be tossed into the washer with towels and they allow for the baby's natural messiness while protecting clothes.) Part of this behavior is related to experimentation and learning—she's trying to discern texture, smelling to help identify new foods, and so on. Your baby is using her fingers to experience new flavors and tastes—to see if it's a familiar food.

The trouble comes when the learning disintegrates into playing in the food (throwing food, rubbing food in hair or clothing). This should be stopped. Simply take the food away and remove her from the high chair. If you do this consistently and reinforce it by telling her that the food is not to play with, she will eventually understand this is not acceptable. Babies can learn even in early months that eating is a serious business and not a play time. You have to put your foot down early; playing with food or using food to get attention can become a serious problem.

Through all this, try to be patient and encouraging. It could be over 18 months before your baby can really feed himself a meal. The attention spans of babies are short, so you'll need to feed him the first bites of foods and finish feeding the last few, even after he has practiced self-feeding. He'll also probably spill more than he eats at first. Don't be overly concerned about tidiness or the use of a spoon or fork until your baby is ready. The prime objective at this point is to be sure he is eating a variety of foods and in the amounts needed for growth. Manners and neatness will come later. We promise.

Special Concerns During the First Year

Overfeeding and Overeating

As foods other than breast milk or formula are eaten in larger amounts, the amount of milk should be reduced (from 32 ounces down to 20 to 24 ounces, etc.) so that your baby doesn't get excessive calories. Overfeeding or allowing overeating at this time may begin a lifelong habit of overeating.

Remember at this age and all others of childhood, you provide the food (what baby eats) and the environment or times for eating, but she determines how much food is eaten. Be attentive to cues from your baby that she has had enough, whether from the bottle or foods. Do not continue to feed or encourage eating after your baby has signaled that she is full or satisfied.

Spitting Up

Overfeeding at single feedings is the most common cause of "spitting up." This should be a signal to reduce the amount of formula per feeding. It's difficult to over feed a breast-fed baby, so nursing mothers report less spitting up.

Sometimes swallowed air or a big burp will cause spitting up. Cradling your baby in your arms on a slant (his head higher than his thighs and feet) with no air space in the bottle near the nipple will prevent him from swallowing air.

Check the hole in the nipple. If the formula runs out in a steady stream, the hole is too large, which allows your baby to gulp formula and air with each suck. The holes in the nipples should be such that the formula drips out one drop at a time. This means he has to suck to get formula.

Feedings that are spit up look large because the milk has already started to digest and may look curdled, resulting in small spots on the "burp cloth." On the other hand, vomiting is made up of large amounts of formula which looks as though it has been digested already. It's usually brought up with some force and can be projected across your lap. When this occurs, you must call the doctor at once.

Weaning: When and How?

"When do I wean my baby?" is a common question of all mothers, whether they are breast feeding, bottle feeding, or a combination of the two. Unfortunately, there's no magic answer. There isn't even a standard or routine answer. Each infant and mother must determine their own schedule. For most infants weaning just comes naturally when the infant decides he no longer wants or needs the sucking and intimacy—usually somewhere around 1 year of age. This is the time when he is developmentally capable of partially feeding himself with fingers and a spoon and drinking from a cup or glass.

Since most of an infant's nourishment comes from breast feeding or a bottle during the first 6 months, weaning should not be done until he is getting adequate milk and food daily from other sources. Infants usually start to eat more food when weaning.

Make sure your baby drinks enough formula or milk after weaning is accomplished. Some infants may resist milk, especially if the bottle or breast is taken away too quickly. Weaning should be a gradual process with preparation and planning.

It's important to provide your baby with experiences that lead to giving up the bottle or breast. For instance, try giving formula or pumped breast milk in a cup as early as 4 months or when he has good head control and sitting balance. Do not make the mistake of only putting juice in the cup because at some point you'll expect him to take milk from the glass as well. Let him adjust to breast milk in a cup as he begins to use a cup.

The change from breast milk or formula to other forms of milk should also be gradual. Mixing the milk of your choice with pumped breast milk or formula and gradually eliminating the breast milk or formula is a good way to get him to accept the new milk and in the quantities needed for adequate nutrition. Some babies will go directly from breast milk or formula to other milks and not miss a beat. If your infant marches to the beat of another drummer, just keep offering small amounts of milk at each feeding. Most children come back to milk (after avoiding it for a time) fairly quickly unless you make such an issue of it that your child uses the situation to manipulate your behavior. During the time your child is not drinking milk, serve other sources of calcium, such as cheeses, yogurt, ice cream, or dark green vegetables.

Obesity

Babies are naturally fat. At no other time does the body have as high a fat-to-lean ratio as during the first year.

If you suspect your baby is "getting too fat," check with your doctor to determine your baby's rate of growth. (More about growth charts in Chapter 3.) If it's significantly faster than normal, it may signal overfat is on the way. Your doctor or a registered dietitian can design a feeding plan to slow the growth rate down, preventing obesity. Do not attempt to decrease the calories in your baby's diet during the first year without seeking professional advice.

Colic, Gas, Fretfulness, Stomach Cramps

There's a disagreement as to whether "colic" exists and, if it does, what is it? Some babies seem to be fussier than others after feeding. Mothers describe "cramping" (feet drawing up), gas (passing foul smelling gas), crying without consolation, and inability to sleep. If your baby has these or any symptoms you think are unusual or abnormal, don't hesitate to call your doctor. Even though this may be colic and not really treatable, these same symptoms could signal other conditions your doctor can treat.

Chapter 3

The Independent Toddler

(12 to 36 months)

Physical Growth and Development

Your life may be getting more hectic, but your toddler is slowing down—his growth, that is. During the toddler years, children grow much more slowly than during the first year. Oh, there will be occasional spurts of growth, but they'll be followed by periods when you think nothing is happening (until you notice his shoes are too small or pants too short).

Changes in height and weight are more subtle in the toddler years than during the first 12 months. As noted in the chart on the next page, toddlers gain an average of 6 pounds a year. That's approximately half the rate of babies less than a year old.

GROWTH EXPECTATIONS
AVERAGE CHANGES IN WEIGHT AND HEIGHT

Age	Weight Gain	Height Gain
0-6 months	1 ounce per day	6 inches
6-12 months	1/2 ounce per day (1 pound per month)	4 inches
1-2 years	1/2 pound per month (6 pounds per year)	4-5 inches
2-5 years	4-6 pounds per year	2-3 inches

During the toddler years, boys and girls have similar growth patterns. Graphs or charts are available from your doctor to compare your child's growth to a standard reference of other children of the same age and gender.

Plotting height and weight over time (two to three times a year during the first 3 years) will show if your child is growing normally or if there may be some problems. But remember, there may be considerable individual differences from one child to another. All 2 year olds are not the same size. And as you probably know, it's impossible to tell how old children are by size. The most common occurrence during these years is that children tend to lose fat and become more lean or slim.

You'll undoubtedly discover that the toddler years are a period of increased physical activity—running instead of walking, and climbing and jumping. Children are eager to try new found muscles. If there are stairs to conquer or a butterfly to chase, they'll do it. Because of this increased activity and differences in body size, the food needs of children must be determined for each individual. How active is the child? How big is his body? Needs are not determined by age or gender.

These years are also characterized by learning, exploring, experimenting, and socializing. All these traits can be used to meet nutritional needs. If you introduce new foods to your toddler, allow her to explore by feeling, tasting, and smelling, and encourage her to eat with her playmates, she'll usually enjoy the foods better.

What Does My Toddler Need?

Meeting the nutritional needs of your toddler will take a little work and careful planning on your part. Note the Food Pyramid on page 115. Toddlers have limited stomach capacity. They cannot eat enough in three meals so they must have nutritious snacks between meals to meet their calorie needs. And because they can be incredibly active, "every bite must count," none should be wasted on low-nutrient foods. Meals and snacks must be planned to complement each other.

DAILY REQUIREMENTS FOR TODDLERS

Meat and meat alternatives	2-3 servings daily (1 serving = 1 ounce)
Fruits and vegetables	5 or more servings daily (1 serving = 2 tablespoons)
Breads, cereals, and grains	6 or more servings daily (1 serving = 1/4 to 1/2 slice)
Milk, yogurt, and cheese	3-4 servings daily (1 serving = 1/2 cup)

How Much Should I Serve?

Children's appetites vary considerably between days and even from one meal to the next, so you shouldn't expect (or demand) a clean plate every meal. It's tough to know how much food you should serve, but a good rule of thumb is 1 tablespoon of each food per year of age. Don't be too concerned that he gets the right amount of nutrients at each and every meal or snack. It's more important that his nutrient needs are met by averaging intakes over time.

The following chart shows the amounts of foods in different food groups that are necessary to meet the nutritional needs of toddlers. If your child is exceptionally active, serve more energy-dense or high-calorie foods. This is true for both boys and girls.

SUGGESTED SERVING SIZES FOR 1 TO 3 YEAR OLDS

BREAKFAST

Milk	1/2 cup
Juice, fruit	1/4 cup
Cereal	1/4 cup
Bread	1/4-1/2 slice

MID-MORNING OR MID-AFTERNOON SNACK

Milk, fruit, vegetable juice	1/2 cup
Bread	1/4-1/2 slice
Graham crackers, 2" x 2"	1
Vanilla wafers	2

LUNCH OR DINNER

Milk	1/2 cup
Meat/meat alternative—	
Poultry, fish, cheese	1 ounce
Cooked egg	1/2 egg
Cooked dry beans or peas	2 tablespoons
Peanut butter	1 tablespoon
Vegetables	2 tablespoons
Fruits	2 tablespoons
Bread	1/4-1/2 slice
(whole grain or enriched)	

What is a Food Jag?

So, your little girl wants a peanut butter sandwich every meal? Welcome to the world of food jags.

The first thing you should know is food jags are normal. Children get in a rut; they want to eat the same foods over and over, sometimes in large quantities. The second thing to know is food jags are usually short-lived. They do not present a problem unless the jag gets excessive attention or causes a disturbance. Your child may try to eat one food, excluding all others, to get her way or to control your behavior.

Of course, no single food contains all the nutrients your toddler needs, so you should keep on offering a variety of foods each day. She'll eventually put down that peanut butter sandwich. If the jag does persist indefinitely, see your doctor.

Toddlers also like to fill up on one food (i.e. milk or bread) and then they do not have room for other foods. Generally, the foods they overeat are very easy to eat (cookies, crackers, bread) or drink (milk, soft drinks, juice, etc.). This problem is usually solved by offering other foods first during meals and spacing meals and snacks at least 1 and 1/2 to 2 hours apart. Also, it might be best to serve beverages after the meal or at least after much of it has been eaten.

Avoiding Food Battles

The attention spans of toddlers are quite short, so it's unrealistic to expect them to sit through family meals that last more than 30 minutes. Eating can quickly turn into playing in food, refusing to eat, throwing food, etc. To avoid this, you may allow your child to eat before the family. But it's important that he later sits for awhile with the family at mealtime.

If your child refuses many foods, he may be more interested in eating if you let him help prepare the foods or set the table. It also helps to place small portions on his plate at one time. Toddlers thrive on attention and praise. They like to finish everything and then ask for more. Unfortunately, adults usually try to put much more food on a child's plate than they can possibly eat. This overwhelms many toddlers making them feel defeated or unable to finish all of the food. They are discouraged from eating any at all.

It's not necessary to "force" your child to eat. In fact, coercing him to eat will merely make him more resistant to eating anything.

There should be enough time between snacks and meals for his appetite to develop. The toddler who snacks or nibbles continuously will never get "hungry" and will not eat well at meals. Approximately 1 and 1/2 to 2 hours between meals and snacks is usually enough to preserve his appetite.

Are naps or relaxation times prior to meals helpful to prevent feeding problems? You bet! Your toddler can be too tired to eat. He may fall asleep in the high chair or at the table. Or become too irritable to be interested in food. When this happens, it's better to put him down for a rest or nap. His appetite will be increased after the rest.

Establishing Good Food Habits and Feeding Skills

Just as your infant is gradually weaned from sucking the bottle to drinking from a glass, your child progresses gradually from spoon to fork and finally to knife and fork for cutting.

Encouraging your child to eat at her current development level will allow her to achieve orderly feeding skills. Be wary of expecting too much; it could cause problems. Toddlers should be encouraged to feed themselves, using their fingers at first and progressing to a spoon. (Be sure to use foods that are suitable for finger feeding or ones that will cling to a spoon.) Fingers foods may be more appropriate for snack foods, while foods requiring utensils may be better for meals.

Correct use of the fork—spearing first and then lifting—comes later at 4 to 5 years. Your child may be 6 to 8 years old before she can use a knife for cutting rather than spreading. Even then, your child must have had an opportunity to practice and experiment. You cannot put a utensil in your child's hand and expect her to be skilled her first try.

Why Doesn't He Like Some Foods?

Is your child a "picky" eater or "particular" about foods? It doesn't necessarily mean he dislikes the food or is misbehaving. Many children reject foods that are difficult to chew; meats are the most common.

It takes time for a child to develop chewing skills. On top of that, there's new teeth, sore gums, and new food experiences to deal with. Your child may chew inadequately and not be able to swallow, and then spit the food out. In many instances the food is not tender or small enough. Because of this, tender meats in small pieces should be the first meats offered.

Unfamiliar textures (crisp, hard, stringy, or lumpy) may also be rejected at first. Children reject more foods on the basis of texture than taste. It's best to offer single food items that can be carefully scrutinized for smell, texture (feeling by hands and in the mouth), and taste. If you serve a mixture, your child may methodically pick familiar items out and leave those he cannot recognize.

You may be amazed at how quickly your child will change his food likes and dislikes during this age and on into the preschool years. A food that has been consistently rejected at home may suddenly be accepted at a friend's house or in a group care setting with peers. Children are great imitators. If mom, dad, teacher, or a friend eats something, your child may be motivated to try it.

DEALING WITH A PICKY EATER

- Don't bribe, punish, or console your child with food. This could lead to a lifetime problem. Food isn't something that should be tied to our emotions at an early age.

- Set good examples. Your child will most likely follow your eating habits.

- Don't offer too many snacks. A hungry child at mealtime will eat more and often try new foods.

- Don't argue with your child while eating or force him to eat any particular food. If he doesn't care for one food, try a nutritional equivalent. Refer to page 89 for some suggestions. Mealtime is not to be used for discipline.

- Let your child fill his own plate from the choices available. Tell him to select at least three items from those offered (i.e., bread, vegetable, potato, fruit).

- Allow your child to help in meal preparation and table setting. Mealtime is often more interesting for children if they help prepare for it.

Introducing New Foods

Mothers frequently ask us, "How can I get my child to try new foods?" This is a valid concern. Children need to appreciate new foods so they can eat a wide variety of foods and adjust to new feeding situations outside the home (such as at a baby sitter's, day care center, or restaurant). Plus, the more foods your child accepts, the better her possibilities to be well nourished.

The best way to teach nutritious food choices is to make nutritious foods available. And this is the parent's responsibility. Once your child learns to choose and like nutritious foods, she will continue to eat them. Just remember to make sure the foods are easy to eat and quickly available to her.

When introducing your child to a new food, remember two key words: explore and experience. Help her develop a positive, curious attitude toward foods. There is much she can learn about a new food before it becomes a favorite or preferred food. Making new foods available on a regular basis helps to develop familiarity and acceptance.

Your child explores and learns with all five senses: sight, touch, smell, taste, and sound. Food can be used to take advantage of those senses. Talk with her about the characteristics of the food that are obvious to see: color and shape.

Next, your child may want to feel the food, using fingers first. Concepts of smooth, hard, rough, sticky, and soft can be stressed as she becomes familiar with the feel of the food.

Before exploring the feel of the food in her mouth, she may want to smell it, which should be encouraged. Many foods are eaten primarily because of their pleasing aroma.

Tasting may offer the most exciting aspect of new food. As new flavors (sour, sweet, salty, strong, mild) are experienced, help your child become aware of the similarities and differences.

How a new food feels in the mouth is also important to a child. For instance, mashed potatoes may be her favorite food and flavor until she tries some "lumpy" potatoes. As we've said, food is often rejected on the basis of texture rather than taste.

Don't forget that foods can make sounds. What better way could there be to learn the full meaning of such concepts as crisp or crunchy? A "noisy" eater may just be having fun with food sounds. Remember the sounds of dry cereal in milk?

Your child should be given opportunities to explore or experiment thoroughly with any new or strange food. Yes, this method of teaching food appreciation may create some "messes" from a parent's viewpoint. But children cannot be made to enjoy a food—they must be *allowed* to enjoy it.

GOOD BOOKS ON EATING HABITS TO READ WITH YOUR CHILDREN

Bread and Jam for Frances, by Russell Hoban, Harper & Row, 1964.

Green Eggs and Ham, by Dr. Seuss, Random House, 1960.

When, What, and Where to Snack?

As mentioned before, toddlers have small stomach capacities and short attention spans. Because of this, it's important to plan more than three meals a day. Between meal feedings or snacks must be as carefully planned as meals in order to meet nutritional needs. Unfortunately, "snacks" mean something other than nutritious to some children and families.

Since your toddler is at the age of "independence," snacks should be easy to handle so he can feed himself. The following is a list of good finger food snacks and between meal feedings.

FINGER FOOD SNACKS AND BETWEEN MEAL FEEDINGS

Meat/protein foods

peanut butter
hard cooked eggs
cold chicken/turkey

Raw vegetables
(plain or with dip)

turnip slices
zucchini slices
green beans
cucumber slices
red/yellow sweet peppers
carrots/baby carrots
tomato wedges
celery sticks stuffed with
    cheese or peanut butter
broccoli florets

Milk/dairy foods

yogurt
cottage cheese
cheese (sticks/cubes)
milk shakes
ice cream, sherbet,
ice milk, frozen yogurt

Fruits

apple wedges
banana slices
strawberry slices
soft dried fruit
peach/pear slices
grapefruit sections
seedless grapes
melon balls or cubes
pitted prunes or plums
cauliflower
raisins/yogurt raisins

Breads/cookies/cereals

bread sticks
pretzels
toasted bagel/pita chips
rice cakes
mini muffins
graham crackers
french toast sticks

animal crackers
oatmeal cookies
raisin bread
mini bagels
vanilla wafers
fruit-filled cookie bars

Toddlers can easily become "nibblers" or "grazers" (eating small bites continuously throughout the day) if they are allowed to eat frequently and constantly all over the house. Your child may even hide a piece of toast in her toy box only to return to it that same day or the next. Of course, this grazing behavior should be left to cows. It's not conducive at all to a toddler eating at mealtime.

You must allow time (1 and 1/2 to 2 hours) between meals and snacks for your toddler to get hungry again. If food and beverages are offered too close together, she will eat less overall. There should be a set time to begin and end snacks as well as a designated place where she can sit—perhaps a small table in her room or the family table. And make sure the table and chairs are set-up appropriately so her feet can rest on the floor, blocks, or telephone books. This gives some balance to an otherwise uncoordinated child.

Preparing for the Preschool Years

Your child's early years are the nutrition preparation period for childhood and adolescence, when his nutritional needs will be greater. The preschool years will be a time of rapid and constant growth for your child, so he'll need an increasing amount of practically all nutrients.

This age is perfect for establishing good food habits because your child is eager to learn and learns well and easily from repetition and experience. These eating habits will play a major role in your child achieving his maximum potential for physical and mental development.

Chapter 4

The Preschool Years

(3 to 6 Years)

Congratulations! You've survived the "terrible twos," those of the independent toddler. The next step in your child's growth is also very dependent on good nutrition. Now's the time when your child begins to establish regular eating patterns and various likes and dislikes that can stick with him for years. It is, of course, especially important that you help your child develop healthy attitudes toward food.

Most likely your child will pay great attention to what you do. He may, in fact, mimic your eating habits. It's at this stage that you can guide your child to healthy eating habits and teach him to make his own choices. This is far better than forcing him to eat or disciplining him during mealtimes. Not only is this frustrating, but it may, in the long run, cause eating problems. Instead, emphasize the fact that eating can be fun and pleasurable.

This is also the time to focus on table manners. Good manners will become habits at an early age and it's best to start children off right so they'll feel comfortable wherever they eat—at home or away.

Your child should not be in charge. It's still up to you to see that his basic needs are met, especially while you continue to control his eating experiences. Once he goes off to school and spends less and less time with you, his eating patterns and food choices are out of your control. If you teach him at home and within the family, he'll most likely continue to make good food choices away from home.

What Does My Preschooler Need?

Again, it's important to emphasize good food choices as outlined in the Food Pyramid on page 115 (i.e., lean meats and protein sources, milk and milk products, fruits and vegetables, and whole-grain enriched breads and cereals). Portion sizes should be a child's size (average of 1 tablespoon per year of age). She can always get seconds if she wants. Large servings tend to discourage eating.

DAILY REQUIREMENTS FOR PRESCHOOLERS

Meat and meat alternatives	2-3 servings daily (1 serving = 1 1/2 ounces)
Fruits and vegetables	5 or more servings daily (1 serving = 1/4 cup)
Breads, cereals, and grains	6 or more servings daily (1 serving = 1/2 slice)
Milk, yogurt, and cheese	3-4 servings daily (1 serving = 3/4 cup)

Probably the most important point to consider is offering those foods that not only meet your child's nutrition needs, but also are in the form or texture that she'll accept. For example, your child may prefer moist foods to dry, or lukewarm food rather than very hot or very cold. Flavors may also make a difference in food acceptance. Most children are sensitive to highly seasoned or off-flavor foods, so it's probably a good idea to skip the curry dishes.

Encourage your child to enjoy foods that can be picked up with the fingers. It gives her a sense of independence. Carrots can be served as carrot sticks or sliced (and they become pennies or wheels). Meats and cheese can be cut in strips or cubes. Broccoli can be served as flowers or trees.

Talk to your child in a way that she notices the shapes you have given these foods. Children usually enjoy comments about their foods that relate to familiar subjects (wheels, pennies, sticks, cubes, flowers, trees). Just remember that the feel of food is important to your child, so if it's slippery or sticky, she may shun it. Make positive comments about the food with a smile on your face as you offer it. A positive approach is the best strategy for establishing good food acceptance.

Preschoolers can follow a similar eating pattern as toddlers, only with slightly larger portions. The following guide is helpful for planning meals for this age group. If your child is exceptionally active, additional foods and amounts can be included.

SUGGESTED SERVING SIZES FOR 3 TO 6 YEAR OLDS

BREAKFAST

Milk	3/4 cup
Juice, fruit	1/2 cup
Cereal	1/3 cup
Bread	1/2 slice

MID-MORNING OR MID-AFTERNOON SNACK

Milk, fruit, vegetable juice	1/2 cup
Bread	1/2 slice
Graham crackers	2
Vanilla wafers	4

LUNCH OR DINNER

Milk	3/4 cup
Meat/meat alternative—	
Poultry, fish, cheese	1 1/2 ounce
Cooked egg	1 egg
Cooked dry beans or peas	1/4 cup
Peanut butter	2 tablespoons
Vegetables	1/4 cup
Fruits	1/4 cup
Bread (whole grain or enriched)	1/2 slice

When Others are Taking Care of Her

As devoted as you are, there are going to be times when a baby sitter, grandparent, or day care provider will care for your child. Someone else may be caring for him for a while, but you need to make sure his nutritional needs are met in your absence.

If your child attends a day care center, investigate the variety of foods that are served, not only to see if your child's nutritional needs are met, but also to avoid repeating the same meals at home. Most approved day care centers have their menus planned by a registered dietitian.

You know your child's needs and his food preferences. Most caretakers want your input because good nutrition will enhance your child's personality and boost his overall performance.

Tell your child's caretaker to keep some form of a feeding schedule. It's important to keep most eating to mealtimes. Snack times should be an opportunity to offer foods that enhance your child's appetite (fresh fruits, cheese sticks, mini bagels). Candies, cookies, and other similar foods do just the opposite.

And keep on encouraging your child to feed himself, especially as he goes through preschool and into kindergarten, so that he continues to develop good eating habits.

Concerns With a Second Child

It's hard on a child when she gets a new brother or sister. She's no longer the only cute kid in the house, and now has to compete for attention. It's especially tough when she sees that the care given the baby has dramatically taken time away from her. It may even cause behavior problems.

When a second child comes along, you must carefully prepare your older child as much as possible for changes in routine. It's also important to show her that she is still loved.

Be sure to include her in as many ways as you can in the care of the baby. For example, at feeding time offer her a snack or meal at the same time.

Your older child may even start imitating the baby and want to nurse. Don't make her feel guilty about this. Rather, create a similar situation for her with a doll or teddy bear and a bottle. Making your older child a viable part of the family is most important and can help to prevent resentment to the baby.

In eating situations, as the baby grows, he will most likely try to imitate his older sister. In ways, this is all right, unless it involves undesirable eating habits. Again, it should be emphasized that disruptive behavior and language are not tolerated at the table, both for the baby and older child. On a more positive note, though, your younger child may feed himself sooner and become more independent in his feeding process as he continues to imitate his older sister.

How Do I Teach Him to Make Wise Food Choices?

Young children are notorious for going through phases, mostly temporary, but frustrating all the same. Many times children reject foods one time but later accept the same food. Or a child may suddenly reject his favorite food—perhaps he grew tired of it because a parent served it too much.

When situations like these occur, it's best to continue offering wise choices, exposing your child to a variety of foods and allowing him to make his own choices. He'll most likely begin to select appropriate foods for himself. Remember that children mimic parents, brothers and sisters, and others. Try to be the best example you can be.

It's important that you try to establish healthy eating habits. Even so, it's OK to take an occasional trip to a restaurant for a hamburger, french fries, cookies, ice cream, etc. But these high fat choices need to be balanced by the remaining meals of the day with lower fat foods such as fruits and vegetables.

Do your best to make mealtime pleasurable; it will make an atmosphere for good acceptance of healthy foods. It's upsetting if foods are rejected—you want the best for your child—but try to remain calm. Children learn very quickly how to push their parent's "button." Your child may even try certain behaviors just to see how you react. So remember, don't coerce—he may become more stubborn. He may even occasionally only eat one item on his plate, but once he's hungry, he'll eat. And eat.

Having a preschool aged child is certainly a challenge, but your best tactic—and your responsibility—is to continue to offer foods that will help him make good choices. On the following page, you'll find a number of wise food choices.

Preschoolers may have strange food preferences, but they also are very curious. Experimenting with foods can be fun, so let them enjoy eating. This will be the beginning of a lifelong enjoyment of foods.

WISE FOOD CHOICES

CHOOSE	FREQUENTLY	OCCASIONALLY	NOT AS OFTEN
Fruits & Vegetables	fresh fruits & vegetables canned fruits (packed in juice) unsweetened fruit juices vegetable juices frozen vegetables canned vegetables (without added salt)	canned fruits (packed in syrup) sweetened fruit juices dried fruits canned vegetables (with added salt)	fried vegetables and potatoes fried corn and potato chips
Breads & Cereals	whole grain breads & cereals enriched cooked cereals (oatmeal) pasta brown rice whole grain crackers rice cakes	presweetened cereals enriched white bread white rice graham crackers vanilla wafers	high fat crackers & cookies
Meat / Meat Alternatives	skinless chicken & turkey fresh or frozen fish tuna packed in water dried beans, peas, legumes peanut butter	eggs beef, hamburger ham, veal, pork, lamb	luncheon meats hot dogs sausage bacon
Milk / Dairy Products	low-fat milk (after age 2) yogurt (without added sugar) cottage cheese hard cheese (cheddar, swiss, muenster) mozzarella	whole milk presweetened yogurt frozen yogurt ice milk processed American cheese	ice cream
Fats / Oils / Etc.	low-fat salad dressing & dips	regular salad dressings & dips margarine mayonnaise	butter cream cheese sour cream pastries / donuts presweetened beverages juice drinks / soft drinks candy

Chapter 5

Health Concerns

You can't do much to protect your child from the occasional scraped knee, runny nose, or upset tummy. But there are plenty of other childhood health concerns—some quite serious—that you can control, especially the ones that relate to food and nutrition.

There's a lot of information out there telling parents about the latest threats to their children's health. Unfortunately, the reports are often inaccurate and, in some instances, could cause harm.

Here we help you sort out the fact from fiction and present the most common nutrition-related health concerns.

How Do I Make Food Safer?

Bacteria just love food. In fact, the little critters love food so much that they'll contaminate almost anything associated with eating, from your plates to your hands. Once eaten, they go directly into the digestive system and can cause a number of illnesses, especially in children. It may be obvious, but it's good to remember that food safety all starts with cleanliness. That means the first thing you should do before handling food is wash your hands thoroughly. Here are some other ways to make food safer:

FOOD SAFETY TIPS

- Wash foods thoroughly before preparation.

- Keep dishes and cooking utensils clean.

- Thaw foods properly in the refrigerator rather than at room temperature.

- Once foods are cooked, keep them at the right temperature to prevent bacterial growth or refrigerate them if they will be served later.

- Reheat leftovers only once before discarding.

- Mixtures of food (chicken salad, potato salad, etc.) should be refrigerated after mixing until eaten. If taken on picnics they should be carried in coolers on ice.

If you doubt the safety of any food, throw it out. Why take a chance? You can't always tell if food is spoiled by how it looks or smells. And it's never a good idea to taste food to determine if it's spoiled. Spoiled or contaminated food can cause serious illnesses in small children, especially if it is accompanied by diarrhea or vomiting that can cause dehydration. Your doctor should be contacted immediately.

What about Pesticides, Preservatives, and Other Additives?

You hear a lot about the dangers of pesticides used on crops and additives in food. Yes, some people are sensitive to these chemicals, and it's best to carefully wash fruits and vegetables to remove any pesticide residues. Still, the foods in your grocery store are generally regarded as safe.

Preservatives protect food in shipment and in markets across the country. This is important because spoilage could cause major health problems and decrease the availability of wholesome food for the public.

As for food additives, they are approved by government agencies which certify them as safe. Fewer and fewer additives are being used to preserve foods or extend their shelf life.

Some children may be allergic to coloring agents or other food additives. Although this is uncommon, if you suspect your child is having a problem with some chemicals in foods (symptoms include itching, hives, redness, diarrhea), see your doctor.

Using a Microwave Safely

What would we ever do without the microwave oven? In this time of fast foods and quick preparation techniques, the microwave has become standard in most homes. Most are so easy to use that many older children use them. Even so, that doesn't mean microwaves aren't dangerous. If your child has access to a microwave, she should be taught safety measures before using it and carefully watched to be sure she follows those precautions.

The biggest concern is to protect your child from burns. Microwave ovens cook foods from the inside out, and the center of food is often much hotter than you think. Serious burns occur from handling the hot food without pot holders or trying to eat the food before it has cooled sufficiently.

When cooking rather than reheating, the containers holding the food will be hotter than the food. Children should be taught to remove items—even plastic dishes—with a pot holder. Metal containers or utensils should not be used in microwaves because they can cause sparking, fires, and even explosions.

MICROWAVE SAFETY TIPS

- Make sure the microwave is sturdy and accessible for older children to use.

- Supervise your child's use of oven until you are comfortable with her use of it.

- Insist your children always wear potholders when removing items from microwave.

- Set aside special cookware for microwave use so incorrect containers are not used.

- Teach children basic first aid measures if burns occur and quick treatment is necessary.

Children aren't the only ones that need to be concerned with using a microwave safely. Moms and dads have to remember that microwaves cook foods from the inside out.

You should be especially careful when heating food for infants. Strained foods, if warmed in the microwave, may be much hotter than they appear. The food should be stirred and allowed to cool before offered to your baby.

Formula in bottles should not be warmed in the microwave oven. The shape of the bottle is conducive to hot spots in the formula which you cannot detect when shaking out a few drops. Oven safety is a serious concern. Major mouth and body burns have been experienced by infants and young children.

The Thin or Underweight Child

Unless there's a medical reason, it's important that you don't restrict the calories in your young child's meals and snacks. It could make him underweight and more susceptible to infections and illnesses. It may even stop his growth.

Children are not little adults, and there's usually no reason why they should go on a diet. Their little bodies need enough calories to maintain normal body weight and growth. They can't eat much food at one time because of their size, but they should eat more frequently than adults, usually five or six times per day.

If your child is underweight, it's up to you (with the help of a registered dietitian, perhaps) to carefully choose foods that meet his needs. Serve high-calorie, high-protein snacks and meals, and use whole milk rather than a lower fat alternative. Fat containing foods should not be restricted because they have 2 and 1/4 times more calories than foods containing only protein and carbohydrates. Some parents think they should restrict the fat in their young child's diet. After all, adults are reducing the fat in their diets to reduce the risk of heart disease. But at this time of your child's life, it's more important that he gets enough calories to grow.

That doesn't mean you should let your child eat continuously throughout the day, though. Many underweight children are "nibblers" and never develop an appetite for meals. There's good news, however. They often eat more food when they have specific times to eat, approximately 1 and 1/2 to 2 hours between feedings.

In addition to all this, your doctor may also suggest a multivitamin supplement for your underweight child. (More information on supplements appears on page 71.)

The Overweight or Overfat Child

Most of us know the potential land mines ahead of many fat children. They're often ridiculed by other children or left out of games. Even adults can make hurtful comments. This can cause an explosion of psychological and emotional problems. Body image may become distorted. Self worth is questioned.

Unfortunately, all of these factors may complicate the fat problem by making your child indulge in food and become less physically active. If left unchecked, your child may keep eating more and more food while getting less and less exercise, and those excess calories will be stored as fat.

Overfat children have a greater likelihood of becoming fat adolescents and then fat adults. In addition to psychological problems, being overfat can result in health problems such as cardiovascular and other chronic diseases. In short, you should not ignore your child's weight problem. First, though, it's most important to understand the concept of overfat or obesity.

Not all overweight children are obese or overfat. Some are heavy because they have more muscle and bone tissue. You merely can't look at a child and determine the degree of fatness. Nor can weight alone indicate obesity. Muscle and fat tests must be done.

If you suspect your child is getting too fat, seek professional help. Ask your doctor if your child is overweight or overfat. Once this determination has been made, a registered dietitian can advise you how to balance your child's diet with physical activity. Weight reduction plans for children must be done carefully because extreme calorie reductions may result in decreased or stunted growth. This is why professional help is critical for initial planning and continuous monitoring over time.

If your child is only slightly overfat, you may be counseled to hold his present caloric intake to maintain a stable weight (stop the gaining) rather than trying to lose weight. In time, his gains in height may better balance his weight.

It would also be helpful to figure out which foods, if any, your child is eating in excess, what times during the day he is eating, and what attitudes may be triggering his overeating behavior. Some fat children do not eat a lot more than their lean peers—they're just a lot less active. A food and activity record may show that your child should increase his daily exercise or physical activities to balance his weight. Incidentally, a food and activity record is beneficial to parents of all children—no matter what their weights.

SAMPLE FOOD AND ACTIVITY RECORD

Time	Food/Beverage Eaten	Activities/Time Spent	
8 a.m.	1 cup cornflakes 1/2 cup milk 1/2 slice toast	sitting at table	15 min.
8:15		walked up stairs put on clothes walked downstairs	2 min. 10 min. 2 min.
8:30			
8:45		outside to swing slide walking/running	5 min. 5 min. 5 min.
9:00			
9:15			

For your child's food and activity record, list each food or beverage he consumes and in what amount—spoons, parts of a cup, or in bites. Be sure to list water, snacks, and other foods eaten between meals. This information will show how much and how often he is eating and the time between meals and snacks. Perhaps you could help to establish better food habits by encouraging him to stay longer at the table or reduce the number and amount of snacks.

His activities and their approximate times should be described. Include naps (lying still, asleep) and nighttime sleeping, TV watching, reading, etc. It's also good to notice what eating behaviors, if any, are associated with activities. (For instance, does he always eat something when he's watching TV?) In a week or less, you'll realize just how active or inactive your child is.

The food and activity record should be kept on the refrigerator or some other easily accessible spot so recordings can be made throughout the day. It's not possible to remember everything at a later time, so write it down as you go. Take the records with you when you go to the doctor to discuss how much your child is eating and how active he is.

Only when foods and activities are recorded can you really know what your child is eating. Most people underestimate food eaten and overestimate physical activity if they rely on their memory. The written record pinpoints problems and opportunities for improvement.

Establishing good food habits and regular exercise for your preschooler will help him form a healthy lifestyle as he becomes an older child and adult. This is especially true since food habits are much easier to *mold* at this time than to *change* as your child gets older. Limit the amount of empty-calorie foods around the house that have no significant nutrients. And get involved with your child in physical activities. Studies have shown that lean parents tend to have lean children.

Cholesterol, Fat, and Heart Disease

There is some evidence that childhood factors (eating habits, for example), along with genes, may contribute to heart disease in later years. Researchers are already fairly certain that heart disease in adults has genetic origins. And obesity, smoking, and high blood pressure will increase a person's risk of heart disease. Now they're trying to determine whether changing (or modifying) food habits—eating less fat and cholesterol—in childhood can decrease the incidence of disease later in life.

This does not mean all fat and cholesterol is bad. In fact, fat is a necessary nutrient for everyone, especially for infants and young children. Fat has an important role in brain development and growth. Therefore, it's suggested that children over 2 years get at least 30 to 40 percent of their total daily calories from fat. (This compares to less than 30 percent of total daily calories for adults.)

Fat intake is not restricted, at all, for children under 2 years.

Calories from fat should be averaged over a day's and week's time because not all foods, snacks, or individual meals can be within the 30 to 40 percent fat range. Some foods have a higher concentration of fat, others a lower concentration. The overall average should be your main concern.

Cholesterol is vital during the early years for development of the body's nervous system, formation of hormones, and as an important structural component of body cells. However, too much cholesterol can lead to risk of heart disease, stroke, or other diseases in later years. Although cholesterol restrictions are not placed on infants and children, you should become aware of products and foods made from animal fats, and avoid using them in excess.

Does your family have a strong history of heart disease or elevated blood lipids (fats)? If so, your children should be screened for fat and cholesterol levels. If they are elevated or abnormal, some complex dietary changes will be necessary, with the guidance of a registered dietitian. Eating habits will need to be changed and continued throughout life.

WHAT IS FAT AND CHOLESTEROL?

Fats are substances made up of various combinations of fatty acids. They can be classified as:

- saturated—those generally solid at room temperature. Saturated fats raise blood cholesterol and are found in animal foods, tropical oils, and hydrogenated oil. (Examples include beef fat, butter, coconut oil, cream, lard, palm oil, shortening, whole milk, and whole milk products, such as ice cream and cheese.)

- unsaturated—those usually liquid at room temperature. Unsaturated fats may help lower blood cholesterol. They are composed of fatty acids that are either polyunsaturated (margarine and vegetable oils from corn, sunflower, safflower, or soybean oil) or monounsaturated (peanut, olive, and canola oil, or avocados.)

Cholesterol is not a fat, but it is a fat-like substance found in fats and oils only in animal products (meat, butter, eggs, milk).

Hyperactivity and Sugar

Does it seem like your child is always "bouncing off the wall" or "can't sit still"? Many moms and dads come to us frazzled and say their child is practically "swinging from the chandeliers" night and day, or (our favorite) has "ants in the pants."

Almost all of them are convinced their child is hyperactive. They say "chocolate sets her off," or "sugar causes him to be nervous or hyperactive."

What they don't realize is that much of what they describe is normal behavior. Children know certain behaviors get a lot of attention. And they can turn those behaviors on and off at will, with or without the help of foods, sugars, or coloring agents.

Part of the confusion of parents may be caused by the fact that there *is* a behavioral disorder known as attention deficit hyperactive disorder (ADHD). However, it only affects a very small percentage of children. Furthermore, scientific evidence does not support a connection between food eaten and ADHD. Studies have shown that sugar does not increase hyperactivity. In fact, sugar has a calming influence on many children. Again, there's no evidence that links the eating of coloring agents or artificial sweeteners to hyperactive behavior.

This points out once again that a balanced diet and a variety of food is desired. If your child consumes excessive amounts of sugar, her appetite is dulled for nourishing foods. Sugar contains only calories—no other nutrient.

Are Sweeteners Bad?

There's a lot of discussion in the media about the safety of sweeteners for children. The most recent controversy is over aspartame (sweetener in NutraSweet®). Although research has shown aspartame is safe for children and does not adversely affect their behavior, it does not contain any nutrients. Aspartame is known as a "non-nutritive sweetener," which means it has little place in the diet of your child who needs nutrients in everything she eats.

What about other sweeteners? Taken in small amounts, low-calorie sweeteners are no problem for children. But again, keep in mind that your child needs to eat a variety of nutritious foods to grow. Lower-calorie products are not appropriate for young children. In fact, the calories from sugar may be necessary to maintain desirable weight. If your child eats too much food with no nutritive value, she will not have an appetite later for nutritious food. Non-nutritive sweeteners, therefore, are recommended only for obese children or for children who have problems with sugar, such as those with diabetes.

Dental Health

There's a considerable relationship between what your child eats and his dental health. Dental cavities (caries) and tooth decay are caused by bacterial action on food residues left on the teeth. Some foods, like sweets and sugar, provide a better medium for cavity-causing bacteria than others. Ideally, you should brush your child's teeth, or at least rinse out his mouth, after every snack and meal to best remove food and decrease the opportunity for cavities to develop.

Eating an adequate variety of nutrients is essential for a healthy mouth. Calcium and fluoride help form strong teeth and vitamin C is important for healthy gums. In addition, foods with textures that require some chewing, like fresh fruits and vegetables, promote good dental health.

Not only does fluoride (whether in food, water, or toothpaste) play a role in the composition of teeth, but it also protects the tooth surface from cavities. One word of caution, however: excessive amounts of fluoride may discolor or mottle the teeth and eventually dissolve some of the tooth structure.

Have you heard about bottle mouth caries? This is a severe condition of decayed teeth when teeth are usually lost in specific arrangements. Bottle mouth caries occur in young children not yet weaned from the bottle. Ordinarily, these children are put to bed or nap with a bottle, usually containing sweetened liquids (but milk is a culprit, too). Because the child sucks in a resting position, the sugar in the liquids sits on the teeth and gums, which causes greater decay. Try to avoid ever starting this habit. Do not put your child to bed with a bottle of any type.

TIPS FOR GOOD DENTAL HEALTH

- Eat well-balanced meals with a variety of foods.
- Limit foods that are high in sugar (candy, pastries, jam).
- Limit foods that tend to stick to teeth (chewy foods, caramel).
- Offer fresh fruits and vegetables frequently because they help clean teeth.
- Brush teeth or rinse after every meal and snack.
- NEVER put your baby to bed with a bottle of any type as this can increased tooth decay.

Exercise and Fitness

Spend even just a little time watching children and you quickly see they have fun doing almost anything. They love crawling, walking, running, or whatever, especially if they're playing with other children and adults. And best of all, they don't even know all the physical activity is good for them. It's FUN to chase a butterfly or crawl after a ball!

Your infant should not spend the entire day in a playpen or crib. Encourage him to expend energy and to develop muscles and coordination. Toddlers like to "perform" or dance to music, roll on a large ball, or ride a tricycle. Before you know it, you'll be chasing after your preschooler as he rides a bicycle with training wheels for the first time. Then there's swimming, skipping rope, and hopping. All these activities should be fun for your child but not continued to the point that he gets overly tired.

The most important thing to remember about exercise for young children is that the activities should be appropriate for their stage of growth and development and not be competitive. If you enroll your toddler or preschooler in organized exercise or physical fitness classes, be sure the instructors are knowledgeable in child growth and development.

TV and video games are the only real threat to exercise at this early age. Seated activities should be monitored and limited if your child begins to consume more calories than he burns. You'll have a good idea this is happening if he's gaining more fat than normal.

Children can learn, even at preschool ages, that there is a relationship between the amount of food eaten and physical activities. This balance must be maintained if desirable body weights are to be achieved and maintained.

ADVANTAGES OF PLAY TIME

- play time is happy time
- it sparks your child's imagination and creativity
- it helps develop social skills and motor coordination
- it begins a lifetime enjoyment of fitness
- play is a child's "work"

Vitamin and Mineral Supplements: Who Needs Them?

Many parents use vitamin and mineral supplements as "insurance policies," particularly if they think their child is not eating enough. Often the supplements are used as substitutes for meals or snacks. Other parents have the attitude that vitamins and minerals are not harmful, so why not?

But all parents should know this: vitamin and mineral supplements will not stimulate appetite or increase energy supply.

Children who eat a variety of foods consistently, from all major food categories—fruits, vegetables, breads, cereals, meats, poultry, and dairy products—do not necessarily need vitamin or mineral supplements. Even children who follow a "vegetarian" diet can get the necessary vitamins and minerals from foods if their meals and snacks are carefully planned. Their parents must have good knowledge of the nutrient composition of foods to be sure that adequate amounts of calcium, iron, and vitamin B_{12} are consumed.

Vitamin and mineral supplements are essential for certain children. Children with any kind of chronic digestive or malabsorption problems must get supplements because they lose more nutrients in their stools than can possibly be replaced by food. These cases are uncommon, though, and these children must generally follow careful food plans directed by doctors and registered dietitians.

If you choose to offer your child a vitamin or mineral supplement, there are many good ones available. Your doctor or registered dietitian can help you select an appropriate supplement. Those at grocery stores, discount stores, and pharmacies are equally good. Just make sure you carefully read the label to determine how much of each vitamin or mineral is provided.

You should also be careful about where you keep the supplements. Children are fascinated by their shapes. Since most supplements taste sweet, young children may think of them as candy. Don't let your child have access to the supply because too many supplements at one time can be very harmful.

Food Allergies

True allergies to foods are very uncommon and involve few foods. Four foods account for most of the allergic reactions in infants and young children—cow's milk, eggs, soy protein, and wheat. You hear a lot about allergies to strawberries, chocolate, and tomatoes, but these rarely cause true allergic reactions. Even with these, many children outgrow the allergy in 3 to 5 years, although some allergies may persist into their adult years.

Children at greatest risk come from families where other members have documented food allergies. If you suspect that your child is reacting to a food, keep a written diary of everything he eats or drinks. Consult your doctor and share your diary of what your child has been eating.

Once a food allergy is confirmed by your doctor, you may want to see a registered dietitian who can help you identify which foods your child will have to avoid. The dietitian can tell you what nutrients he'll be missing, help you make appropriate food substitutions, and tell you if a vitamin or mineral supplement is necessary.

Choking on Foods or Liquids

Young children can choke on any liquid that "goes down the wrong way." Coughing, which follows, usually clears the airway very quickly—in seconds.

Complete blockage of the airway occurs when solid food becomes lodged in the voice box. This can be serious because it may cut off oxygen to your child's body in 1 to 2 minutes. Children are likely to panic because they cannot get their breath and are afraid. Coughing should be encouraged. At the same time, call for emergency help. Do not give the child anything else to eat or drink because it will further block the airway.

Foods that present the greatest risk for choking are hot dogs, wieners, popcorn, tough meat, small hard candies (mints, jaw breakers, etc.), grapes, and saltine crackers. These foods should be chopped in small pieces. Instruct your child to chew well before swallowing.

Peanuts, popcorn, and seeds are small enough to be swallowed whole. If your child chokes or coughs while eating these, they may go into the lungs and cause significant problems. Therefore, these foods are not recommended for children under 5 years of age.

WAYS TO PREVENT CHOKING HAZARDS

- Teach young children to thoroughly chew their food.
- Insist that your children eat while sitting up.
- Don't leave children alone while eating.
- Don't allow your child to stuff too much into his mouth at one time.
- Remove any pits or bones from foods.
- Avoid serving the following foods to children under 5:

  whole hot dogs/wieners
  popcorn
  hard candy
  nuts
  grapes

Chapter 6

Smart Shopping

Does Advertising Influence My Child's Food Choices?

It's no secret that young children know a great deal about foods from TV commercials. Unfortunately, it's the "sugar-coated cereal in fun shapes!" they know about. Have you ever seen a "broccoli—it's good for you" commercial? The more television children watch, the more they will be drawn to advertising. For the most part, foods are not advertised on the basis of their nutritional value, but rather on factors totally unrelated to food such as fun, adventure, favorite cartoon characters, and toys offered by the manufacturer.

Manufacturers are notorious for using whatever advertising strategies attract your child to their products. Children learn to recognize labels and logos, sing jingles and slogans, and identify specific products by their "spokes-characters." When children see these advertisements on their TV screen, it suggests to them that these items are appropriate to eat.

Never before have we faced so many child-oriented products. The children's food market has exploded in the past 5 years. In addition to the cereals—a product category long popular with children—there are bite-sized crackers and cookies, juice boxes, microwavable meals, frozen dinners, and treats. The convenience of many of these meals and snacks has made them appealing to parents, too. Parents can also be sold products through TV as well as popular magazine advertisements.

Manufacturers begin drawing us to their products and winning sales as early as we begin to buy baby foods. To look at a grocery shelf of baby foods alone can be mind boggling. There are first foods, strained, graduates, finger foods; wholesome, mixed, and natural ones; and those with no preservatives.

As for other foods, we tend to buy child-oriented, bite-sized animal crackers, graham crackers, and vanilla wafers; alphabet- and animal-shaped pasta, and pre-sweetened cereals because they appeal to children's imagination and taste buds. Your child might love these products made just for him, but keep in mind, in most instances you'll pay more for these pre-packaged children's foods. If you're watching your budget and prefer to avoid pre-packaged foods, use a little creativity and time to make your own bite-sized or animal-shaped cookies and snacks.

Fortunately, as parents and other consumers become nutritionally aware, food manufacturers are beginning to offer more healthful choices. And they're providing our younger generation with an increasing number of good nutrition messages. The American Dietetic Association and its state affiliates have responded with public service announcements and good nutrition literature. This association and its National Center for Nutrition and Dietetics have designated March each year as National Nutrition Month, which focuses on good nutrition messages for the public. Fast food establishments and various food manufacturers also have become a part of promoting good nutrition during this time.

Food Labels: What Should I Look For?

Some of the most important food messages are found on food labels. Hopefully, you're already reading food labels to try to gauge the impact of product ingredients—notably calories, fat, and cholesterol—on your own diet. Now it's your turn to read food labels to keep track of your child's nutrition.

You've learned that children who have high-fat, high-choles-
terol, or high-sugar diets have increased incidence of tooth decay,
obesity, and heart problems in later years. Try not to be overly
restrictive, but know what your child is eating, especially during
this time when you still have responsibility and influence.

Knowing what foods to select for your child is a challenge in
itself without the added confusion of interpreting nutrition
labels. Years ago labels listed only the product's name. Then, as
more products were introduced and more people became knowledgeable about the benefits of nutrition, labeling expanded.
Unfortunately, it also became more complicated. The Nutrition
Labeling and Education Act of 1990 helped end some of the confusion, though. It requires a standardized label format that allows
consumers to make direct comparisons of nutrient content from
one product to another. In addition, labels are easier to read and
nutrition terms more understandable.

In 1989, several government agencies began cooperative
efforts to reform the existing food labeling system with regulations that would create uniform labeling for virtually all food
products. Their ultimate goal was to:

• take confusion out of reading nutrition labels;
• help consumers select healthier diets, and;
• assist food manufacturers in improving nutritional qualities of
  their products.

Beginning in 1993, food labels are more "reader friendly."
Under the heading "Nutrition Facts," they include information
on nutrients related to today's current health issues:

• total calories   • calories from fat
• total fat   • saturated fat
• cholesterol   • sodium
• total carbohydrates   • dietary fiber
• sugars   • protein
• vitamin A   • vitamin C
• calcium   • iron

Nutrition facts		
Serving size ½ cup (114g)		
Servings per container 4		

Amount per serving		
Calories 260	Calories from fat 120	

		% Daily Value*
Total Fat 13g		20%
Saturated Fat 5g		25%
Cholesterol 30 mg		10%
Sodium 660g		28%
Total Carbohydrate 31 g		11%
Sugars 5g		
Dietary Fiber 0g		0%
Protein 5g		

Vitamin A 4%	Vitamin C 2%
Calcium 15%	Iron 4%

*Percent (%) of a Daily Value are based on a 2,000 calorie diet. Your Daily Values may vary higher or lower depending on your calorie needs:

Nutrient	2,000 Calories	2,500 Calories
Total Fat	Less than 65g	80g
Sat. Fat	Less than 20g	25g
Cholesterol	Less than 300mg	300mg
Sodium	Less than 2,400mg	2,400mg
Total Carbohydrate	300g	375g
Fiber	25g	30g

1g Fat = 9 calories
1g Carbohydrate = 4 calories
1g Protein = 4 calories

Nutrition information on other nutrients is required only when a food is fortified (nutrients are added to a food), enriched (nutrients are restored to refined grain products after they are removed during processing), or a health claim is made about the food.

Ingredient labels are required to appear on all foods that contain more than one ingredient and must list foods in descending order by weight.

Some exceptions to the overall labeling system are allowed. For example, labels existing on products targeted to children under 2 may not carry information on fat content. As we've talked about, fat is important in the diet of babies under 2 years to ensure proper growth and development. If information on fat was outlined, some parents may look at it as being in excess of their child's needs. By the way, unsalted or unsweetened on baby food labels refers to taste rather than nutrient content.

As the nutritional content of foods becomes more important to us and the food labeling system becomes easier to understand and use, more efforts will be made to educate consumers on the best food choices for their particular needs. Education is the key to becoming more aware of what we eat and its nutritional consequences. If you and your child understand the system, then your child will grow up with a broader knowledge of food and food selections. Each generation, then, will follow with a little more information than the one before.

I Dread Trips to the Grocery Store

Sometimes you'll have no choice but to take your child along food shopping. Children look at this as an adventure, but tired and frustrated parents may not feel the same. Many parents resort to feeding their child throughout the store or give in to her request for certain products just to make shopping quicker.

Don't be surprised if your child's favorite cereal and snacks, juice boxes, and candies seem to jump into your shopping cart. They're often purchased without hesitation and sometimes without realization. After your child realizes how rewarding and fun food shopping can be, she'll demand the same treats every time. But you can avoid this trap. Start by telling her that you are not at the supermarket to eat. Make the trip as pleasant as possible, and make it educational.

The best time to shop, especially with children, is after a meal when you and your child are not hungry. If snacking in the store is unavoidable, stick with an apple, banana, raisins, or a bagel; don't grab a candy bar.

Ask your child to help you put foods into the cart or select light-weight items from the shelf. When children help you, they're more likely to forget about satisfying themselves or eating at all. Ask her to choose which fruit for snacks, which vegetables for dinner, which shape of pasta, or flavor of ice cream or ice milk. Children are more interested in eating what they have helped to select.

Shopping becomes a learning experience when you compare brand name products with generic items, and package sizes. Older children will begin to recognize "best buys" if you educate them along the way.

Before you shop, be sure to make a list of what you need. Clip coupons, too, but only for the items you normally use. Sometimes a generic or store brand may even be a better buy than the brand name product with a coupon—COMPARE the savings.

If you need help comparing the savings between products, use the unit price tag. Supermarkets place these labels on their shelves (usually below the food item) to make it easier for you to compare prices. As shown by the following example, the unit price tag indicates the brand name, product description, package size, retail price, and unit price (price per ounce, pound, pint, or number in the package). By comparing prices based on unit price, you can select the best value for your money.

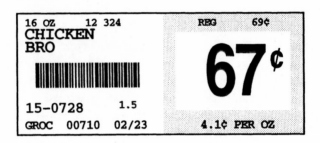

When it's time to leave, look for special check-out lanes without displays of candy or snack items that tempt children. Supermarkets across the country are beginning to come to the aid of parents by providing several aisles of this type. If your supermarket does not have this alternative aisle, talk to the manager about the possibility of opening one.

PUSH A SMART CART—BUY...

- lots of fresh fruits and vegetables
- milk, cheeses, cottage cheese, and yogurt
- lean ground beef, chicken, turkey, and fish
- frozen yogurt and ice milk
- unsweetened breakfast cereals
- mini rice cakes, bagels, and pretzels
- deli-sliced or shaved turkey breast and lean roast beef
- whole wheat or mixed grain breads

Chapter 7

Eating Away From Home

Evaluating Group and Day Care Nutrition: How Do They Rate?

Who feeds your child when he's away from home? What's served? How much time is provided for meals? Are snacks available? How clean and sanitary is the food preparation area? Are the facility and its employees inspected regularly by health authorities? How much food and what kinds will you have to provide from home? Are menus posted?

These are questions that you must ask when your infant or young child spends time away from home. You must continue to monitor these items over time, not just when your child is enrolled. Visit during meal or snack time. See for yourself the interaction of children and staff.

An important aspect is how much time your child is away from home during the day. For some children, this accounts for the majority of their waking hours. Many children consume 90 percent of their nutrients away from home. Therefore, the food served is of major importance to your child's health and nutritional status.

Centers that provide group feeding should be regulated by health authorities for cleanliness and sanitation. Inspection reports are public information and should be posted for you to read. You may feel silly, but it's a good idea to watch the hand washing practices of the person who prepares and serves the food. Food-borne illnesses are frequently transmitted from the person preparing the food to the child, not from child to child.

How are leftovers handled? Are they served again? Leftover foods should be refrigerated or frozen and never reheated for service more than once.

Menus should be posted. Many centers have meals and snacks planned by registered dietitians with experience in child nutrition. Do the menus correspond with the food being served or do they merely decorate the walls? Keep a copy of the menu at home so you can supplement food items that are not being served.

Observe the food habits being encouraged. Are manners and neatness stressed at the expense of eating? Children learn quickly from other children, which can be both bad and good. Your child will pick up habits you may not want, as well as those that are desirable.

Are foods and nutrition education a part of the daily planned activities? Good food and health habits are easily taught at this age and should be part of the educational program. The children should be involved in some simple food preparation activities.

The key is keeping in touch. Know what your child is eating and in what environment. Both are critical to your child's health and nutritional status, now and for the future.

Restaurant Choices

As you may know already, eating at a restaurant with your child can be more of a challenge than a treat. Is it even worth the effort and expense, you ask?

But think about it, eating out is not always a fun thing to do from a child's standpoint, too. It usually means sitting in an uncomfortable chair for a long time and enduring more scoldings about behavior than usual. And, to top it off, your child may not enjoy eating what may be unfamiliar food, even if you order what he wants. Mashed potatoes with gravy or excess butter may not be what he's used to at home. Still, when you do eat out, try the following:

- Select informal family-style restaurants or pancake/waffle houses with efficient service where children are welcome and comfortable. Upscale restaurants probably should be avoided, except with older children.

- Plan mealtimes that best suit your child. You may have to alter your preferred mealtime to better accommodate your child's needs.

- Make sure the restaurant can accommodate your seating preference (i.e., high chair, extra booth space, non-smoking section).

- Ask for a children's menu. If one isn't available, ask for items such as a cheese sandwich or plain hamburger—even if they're not listed on the regular menu.

- Let children share a meal. One adult meal, sometimes even one child's meal, can serve two small appetites nicely. Most restaurants allow you to take home "doggy bags" of food to eat later. This is a better option than insisting that your child eat it all at one sitting.

- Never force your child to try a new food when you eat out. Offer new choices to him from your plate, but don't insist that he eats them. You may set yourself up for an unpleasant scene (and not-so-kind looks from your dining neighbors).

- Be sure to ask how foods are prepared. Your child may not like the butter piled on pancakes, dressing poured over salad, or cheese sauce on steamed broccoli. Request condiments, dressings, and sauces to be served on the side so your child can add them as desired.

- Ask that beverages be served with the meal rather than before. Children tend to fill up on drinks before they have a chance to eat.

- Make a game out of waiting for your meal. If the restaurant doesn't have crayons or coloring materials to keep your youngster busy, take a pen and paper to play dot-to-dot, tic-tac-toe, or drawing and spelling games.

Young children allowed to experiment with various restaurants learn appropriate behavior early on and are likely to be much better behaved at restaurants when they are older.

What About Fast Foods?

Like it or not, convenience and low cost make fast foods an integral part of today's lifestyle, and a popular meal choice of children. The National Restaurant Association says that when children under 17 eat out, they eat at fast food restaurants 80 percent of the time.

Children are attracted to fast food restaurants by catchy advertising and enticing surprises and toys given away with children's meals. Birthday party programs and play areas also help fast food restaurants bring in more parents and children. After all, finding a place for both a low-cost meal and some activity or exercise is very appealing to parents of young children, especially in cold winter months.

Although popular fast foods do provide protein, carbohydrates, vitamins, and minerals, they may be high in fat, sodium, calories, and largely void of vitamin C and fiber.

One way to get a balanced diet is to compensate for the nutritional shortcomings of fast food by serving healthy, well-balanced foods at the remaining meals of the day.

It also helps to make smart choices at the restaurant. Order hamburgers with lettuce and tomatoes; roast beef or turkey sandwiches rather than bacon cheeseburgers; pizzas with fresh vegetable toppings rather than pepperoni or sausage; baked potatoes or coleslaw rather than french fries; and milk or juice rather than soft drinks. Choosing fast foods wisely will teach your child to make better selections, and that's an important education that can last a lifetime.

Children usually go for a traditional child's meal with a hamburger, cheeseburger, or chicken nuggets, french fries, soft drink, and a toy (many times the only reason they want the meal). You can make your child's meal more nutritious by selecting more healthful items from the menu and buying the toy separately. This compromise can make you and your child happy.

Fast food restaurants have responded to consumers' growing nutrition awareness by offering more healthful choices such as broiled chicken and fish, skinless chicken and low-fat hamburgers, and salad bars with options such as cottage cheese, tuna, fruit, and pasta. Many restaurants have even changed their frying source from beef fat to vegetable oil.

In addition, several fast food corporations have registered dietitians on staff and have worked with The American Dietetic Association.

Nutrition information is usually available from fast food restaurants upon request. You should be an informed consumer, knowing your options and those that are best for your children.

Visit fast food restaurants occasionally as a treat, but don't make them a weekly habit. Remember to balance your meals eaten away from home with at-home meals for the best variety and nutrition.

Bag Lunches, Picnics, and More

Your child can learn sensible, healthy eating habits at home. But all that can go out the window once she goes off to school or camp, or off with friends, where you no longer have control over the eating experience.

Even the most carefully planned bag lunch or picnic lunch may be given away or thrown out. When you prepare a carry-out meal for your child, try to pack well-balanced, nutritious foods, as well as ones that are considered more "socially acceptable" to your child. Although she may eat cottage cheese and yogurt at home, that doesn't mean she'll eat them at school. When children are teased about certain foods, they just won't eat them in front of other children. On the other hand, your child may eat foods away from home that she would never eat at home, solely because all her friends are eating them.

Consider your child's preferences, lunch setting, and friends when putting together a camp, school, or picnic lunch. A well-balanced lunch should include a high-protein food, fresh fruit or vegetable, bread or starch, a treat, and milk or juice.

Although sandwiches are traditional lunch choices, other high-protein options include turkey or chicken slices or nuggets, meatloaf, hard boiled egg, and cheese sticks.

If you do go with a sandwich, instead of using bread, try rice cakes, pita bread, tortilla, muffin, bread sticks, bagel, or raisin bread. Your child may even enjoy cooked pasta salad served in a Ziploc® bag. Try tasty and nutritious sandwich combinations such as peanut butter and banana, apple, or finely grated carrot instead of peanut butter and jelly. Cut sandwiches in small (1/4) pieces or strips for easy handling; or be creative by using various cookie cutters to create sandwiches in the shape of hearts, stars, or even Mickey Mouse.

Fruit and vegetable selections could include cherry tomatoes, baby carrots, broccoli florets, applesauce, or slices of cucumber, pear, peach, banana, or pineapple.

For treats, select oatmeal-raisin or peanut butter cookies, or lower-fat foods such as graham crackers, pretzels, vanilla wafers, or presweetened cereal. And little notes, stickers, or cartoons in a lunch bag are a special touch (XXXOOO from MOM). Your child will look forward to a packed lunch if it includes a special surprise.

Chapter 8

Fun with Food

Teaching Children About Food

As we've said all along, children who learn good eating habits tend to be better eaters and better able to select nutritious meals for themselves in later life. Much of this early learning comes from you, the parent. When you make healthy, responsible choices with your own meals and snacks, chances are your child will follow in your footsteps.

Of course, not everyone likes the same foods. Most parents offer their favorite foods to their children, but these choices may not be to their liking. For example, you may like broccoli only with cheese sauce, but don't assume your child will like it that way, too. It's important to give your child a choice. But don't set yourself up for arguments by leaving too many options. Offer two selections, then be creative. (More on being creative later in this chapter.) Although it can take a lot of trial and error, you'll learn eventually what foods he likes most.

The more opportunities your child has to experiment with various foods, the more likely he'll enjoy food. A child who is fed in a loving environment is more likely to enjoy the experience. Children fed with force or impatience, however, tend to develop a negative attitude toward food. Sharing your negative opinions about certain foods in front of your child ("I can't STAND Grandma's tuna casserole.") influences him to reject those foods as well.

It's up to you to give your child a variety of foods. Offering tasty, nutritious options early on teaches your child to appreciate good foods.

WHEN OFFERING NEW FOODS

- Don't force or bribe your child to eat a new food.

- Set good examples by serving everyone the same foods and by eating these foods yourself.

- Offer new foods at the beginning of the meal, when your child is the most hungry.

- Present new foods with at least one food your child likes.

- Don't overwhelm your child with large portions. Start small and let him ask for more.

- Make mealtime a pleasant and relaxing experience, with light and enjoyable conversation—not a time for discipline.

Most children go for plain foods, and prefer raw, crunchy foods over cooked items. Sometimes it's smarter to serve raw carrot sticks or raw fresh green beans rather than a cooked version. Your child may prefer vegetables like broccoli or cabbage raw since they have strong, unpleasant odors when cooked. Children tend to prefer foods served at room temperature. It's also a good idea to use smaller plates and child-sized utensils.

Children like variety in colors, shapes, and textures. For example, baked chicken, carrot sticks, and broccoli florets on a brightly colored plate are more appealing than baked fish, mashed potatoes, and yellow squash on a white plate. Add garnishes of green pepper slices, sliced cherry tomatoes, cantaloupe balls or grapes to entice your youngster's palate. Colorful garnishes please older palates, too.

Don't worry if your child wants a non-traditional food such as pizza or meatloaf in the morning and cereal at dinnertime. Are there really any rules about when foods must be eaten? Although you may become frustrated if these requests happen frequently, you might avoid a confrontation by naming one day of the week to flip-flop meals.

If your child doesn't like or eat a certain food, look for a nutritional equivalent. Some substitutes are listed in the following chart.

NUTRITIONAL EQUIVALENTS

If your child doesn't like...	Try instead...	Why?
meat	eggs, poultry, fish, peanut butter, beans	not as tough and difficult to chew; also good protein source
green vegetables	orange vegetables: carrots, squash, corn, sweet potatoes, beets	not as bitter tasting; comparable nutrient value
any vegetables	fruit: apple, banana, pears, grapes, cantaloupe, watermelon	comparable nutrient value
milk	yogurt, cottage cheese, pudding, flavored (chocolate, strawberry) milk	also good calcium source

You can also include various nutritious foods in favorite meals, such as chopped spinach or sweet pepper on a pizza, and milk in soup, meatloaf, or scrambled eggs. Try new vegetables and various types of legumes in stews and casseroles. Not only do they add to the taste, they also increase nutritional value.

SET SOME HOUSE RULES

- One new food is introduced at dinner on Monday nights.
- You don't have to eat it all, but you have to taste at least one bite. (Remember, a child's bite is smaller than yours.)
- Everyone, parents and children, has the same food on their plates.

Offering foods from other cultures or countries is a good way to teach your child about different ethnic groups. You may be surprised at the new favorites you'll find on a trip to an ethnic market. Your child can also learn about various foods by helping you plant and care for a sprout or vegetable garden. Children love to watch plants grow, especially if they care for them daily, help pick the ripe fruits and vegetables, and sample their own creations.

It's also instructive to take children on trips to farms or orchards and on walks in the country. Seeing chickens lay eggs and cows being milked, and picking apples and berries teaches children about where food comes from and piques their interest in learning.

The importance of safety can also be taught to your child while he is eager. The preschool years are the ideal time to teach him how to use a microwave oven, hot appliances, knives, and special utensils.

Young children can even get involved in following recipes and collecting cookbooks. You should help your child organize ingredients and use the oven, but let him measure, pour, and mix batters. As he grows and develops, more and more can be done independently.

Creating Foods and Menus that Appeal to Children

With a little creativity, mealtime can be fun for everyone, especially when children have a chance to participate. Children learn from doing and they enjoy creating.

- Use cookie cutters to make sandwiches into shapes. Unused bread can be made into bread crumbs for later use or fed to the birds. You can also cut square slices of cheese into shapes. Use leftover cheese in casseroles and for snacks.

- Let your child decorate sandwiches with raisins, apples, banana slices, or grapes. It's amazing how quickly these sandwiches are eaten. Be prepared to make seconds!

- Plain ice cream cones make a nice alternative to bread. Try scooping chicken/tuna salad or cottage cheese into a cone and top with a cherry tomato or grape.

- Pizzas are fun. Spread tomato or spaghetti sauce on uncut pita or English muffins and decorate with mozzarella cheese, green peppers, olives, pepperoni, and mushrooms. Make faces or animal shapes with the cheese and vegetables. Try fruit pizzas, too. (Cut up fruit and decorate over a layer of cream cheese, custard, or pudding.)

- Why not make meatloaf in muffin pans for a change? Top each meat-muffin with a scoop of mashed potatoes and an olive, sliced cherry tomato, or some green peas. Try meatballs served on popsicle sticks. Your child will eat them as though they are lollipops.

- Use child-sized dinnerware, utensils, and placemats. A placemat that's special to a child may depict a favorite character, holiday, or special setting. Help your child make a placemat that displays an actual table setting—plate, glass, utensils, and placemat design. You'll be amazed at how quickly he'll learn to set the table when using this guide.

- Flavored milks or instant breakfast drinks are nice options for children who refuse to drink white milk. Add fruit or chocolate flavors or beverage mixes to milk at half strength to avoid too sweet a taste.

- Serve occasional meals on brightly colored paper plates or ones that illustrate your child's favorite character. Different straws can also add a fun touch to a meal.

At birthday parties, when entertaining your child's friends, have fun with food. Children can wear aprons and dive into spreading fresh vegetables on pizza, skewering fresh fruits on kabobs, and decorating cupcakes—even cupcakes baked in flat bottomed ice cream cones. These activities can be as much fun as hired entertainment—and they cost a lot less.

How Can I Get Him to Help in the Kitchen?

Anything you do in the kitchen looks like fun to your child. Even washing dishes involves bubbles. Children love to help and quite often offer their assistance. Sure, you probably can prepare, serve, and clean up meals quicker and easier by yourself. But what you consider work, your child may consider fun. Allowing children to help makes them feel they've contributed something to the meal. (Plus, children like to eat what they create!)

Helping in the kitchen teaches children skills and techniques important for their lifetime. Children as young as 2 can help in the kitchen with meals and preparing foods. Learning measuring techniques, following recipes, preparing food, and setting a table add to children's math, reading, and social skills and to the development of good manners.

The best part about being involved for your child is his sense of achievement and accomplishment. Younger children can help with tasks such as tearing lettuce, snapping green beans, washing fruits and vegetables, placing bread in baskets, folding napkins, clearing plates, and wiping the table. Older children can measure ingredients, mix batters, husk corn, fill water glasses, butter bread, set the table, and help wash dishes.

Make a game out of preparing, serving, and cleaning up after meals by creating a special day for little helpers and marking it on the calendar. Once the job is complete, place a star or sticker on that particular day. When the month is complete, see how many stars and stickers have accumulated.

For those busy days when you don't want any help in the kitchen but your child is eager and ready, try the following suggestions to keep her entertained:

- Keep a low kitchen drawer filled with coloring/drawing books and crayons for quick, creative art projects.

- Store safe kitchen utensils (wooden spoons, measuring cups and spoons, and plastic containers) in a place where your child can reach them and pretend to cook meals.

- Ask her to fold napkins for future use.

- Let her be creative with food items by stringing macaroni on yarn for necklaces, coloring faces on paper plates, or filling containers with dried beans for a play musical instrument.

Sharing precious time and pleasant experiences with your child in the kitchen creates wonderful memories that last a lifetime. Enjoy them before the time gets away from you.

Creative Birthday and Festive Party Ideas

Children love everything about parties. They love to attend, host, and prepare for parties, whether elaborate family holiday parties, casual birthday parties, or simple tea parties. Several creative party ideas are outlined here:

Animal Safari Hunt

Invitations: Use illustrations or pictures of various animals in a maze-type drawing, stating "Let's Hunt for the Animals."

Activities: Go to a zoo, petting zoo, or farm and hunt for the animals. Stickers could be given to children as they find various types of animals.

Refreshments: Cakes, ice cream, frozen yogurt, or other treats could be decorated with plastic animals or animal crackers.

Nature Hike or Garden Party

Invitations: Create a flower/planter invitation, even including a packet of seeds illustrating the theme, "Come Grow with Me."

Activities: Give everyone a small flower pot, dirt, and seeds to grow their own flower or vegetable plant.

Refreshments: Serve a picnic, including fresh vegetables and fruits, on flowered paper plates and table cloth. Be sure to discuss where various foods come from.

Formal Dress-up Party

Invitations: "Have Tea with Me" invitations could be cut in the shape of tea cups. Be sure to mention that children should wear their favorite dress-up clothes.

Activities: Parade or dance to children's music. Take pictures of the children in their "formal attire." Pin the Cup to the Tea Pot (a version of Pin the Tail on the Donkey) could be played with the children making their own tea cups or bringing their invitations to use.

Refreshments: Serve mini-sandwiches, mini-muffins, or tea cakes with punch or fruit juice "tea" in a child's tea set.

Paint Party

Invitations: Artist palette cut-outs with a paint brush attached create the theme, "Come Paint the Town."

Activities: Use water colors or finger paints to create original art-work. More elaborate activities could include painting shirts with fabric paints. For younger children, it may be more appropriate to use paint-with-water books or paint patios, decks, and out-door furniture with water.

Refreshments: Children can decorate their own cookie or cup-cake with various colors of frosting and toppings. They can also add flavorings (chocolate, strawberry, banana) to milk.

Fun Food Crafts

There are many ways to use foods around the house to be cre-ative. You and your child can enjoy many hours learning about different foods while creating fun, innovative projects. Several simple ideas are listed here:

Pasta Necklaces and Bracelets

Color various pasta shapes with food coloring in water. (Don't soak pasta more than 1/2 hour.) Dry on wax paper. Turn to pre-vent sticking. When dry, cover with acrylic spray. String maca-roni or mostaccioli noodles on yarn.

Picture and Refrigerator Magnets

Follow the previous procedure to color various pasta shapes (shells, wheels, bow ties, spirals) and glue to cardboard. Display as picture or attach magnet to back.

Shakers

Place dried beans or peas in empty gallon milk jug or yogurt con-tainer. Tape tops back on. These make great props for children to dance with.

Bird Feeders

String round breakfast cereals with holes on pipe cleaners. Secure both ends and hang on tree. Also roll empty toilet paper roll in peanut butter and then in bird seed. Punch a hole in the side of the roll and attach a pipe cleaner for hanging onto a tree.

Special Straws

Cut shapes (circles, hearts) from paper plates and decorate. Punch holes in top and bottom of shape and thread straws through holes. It's amazing how special straws make "unfavorite" beverages taste better.

Homemade Play Clay

Use 2 cups flour, 1 cup salt, 2 cups water, 4 teaspoons cream of tartar, 2 tablespoons oil, and 2 drops food coloring. Put all ingredients in pot. Cook and stir constantly over medium heat, until the mixture is the thickness of mashed potatoes. Remove from heat and roll into a ball. Knead with additional flour on waxed paper. Cool and store in airtight container or Ziploc® bag.

Chapter 9

Developing a Healthy Lifelong Foodstyle

How Do I Get the Whole Family Involved?

Mealtimes are more than just eating times—they are family times, happy times for young children and their parents, ones that will be remembered for years to come. Conversation and sharing are a large part of the family meal.

In today's rushed and hurried world, it may be difficult to have every meal be a family meal, but one meal a day (or three to four times a week) should be for the family. The whole family doesn't have to be present, but those that are home should eat together. More families are returning to the old-fashioned, relaxing family dinner. These precious times together help bring a sense of identity to your family, improves communication, and brings closeness to the family atmosphere. Family dinnertime is time to:

- share information about family members, including young children;
- enjoy the company of your family in a relaxed atmosphere while enjoying yourself;
- discuss light topics of interest to everyone;
- focus on family closeness and conversation, not on foods eaten or foods not eaten;
- allow your child to discuss his interests and daily activities;
- listen and talk to your children without criticizing them;
- enjoy nourishing food to satisfy hunger, not to use food as a reward or punishment.

Setting a Good Example

We can't say it enough—the most important way to influence your child's behavior at mealtimes is to set a good example and be a good role model. Your child is a reflection of you. She'll learn to eat by watching you. If you're involved in the meals, and select and eat nutritious foods, she'll want to follow your example.

Children start to note your behaviors and habits at a very young age, and they begin to mimic them immediately. Manners, in addition to eating patterns, are watched constantly. Be prepared for your child to mimic everything, even some things you never realized you did.

Setting Schedules

Meals and snacks should be planned for specific times. Small children cannot go longer than 1 and 1/2 to 2 hours between meals, so meals should be scheduled appropriately. Sometimes six small feedings are most appropriate for toddlers. Once mealtimes are established, try to stick with them. Children need consistency from day to day, but a little flexibility won't hurt. Don't force your child to eat if she isn't hungry, and don't make her wait until she's starving.

Keep in mind that children do not understand the concept of time—they do not know how long one hour is. If your child is hungry and dinnertime is a short time away, explain this time as "when the TV show is over," or "when Daddy gets home," or "when the sun has gone down."

Getting your child on an eating schedule all starts with breakfast, an important part of every child's day. It supplies the nourishment necessary to carry her through an active morning. Because children have not eaten since the night before, at least 8 to 12 hours earlier, their bodies' supply of blood sugar has dropped. Skipping breakfast will cause children to continue to have low blood sugar, and they'll become restless, irritable, and tired before noon. (It can have the same effect on adults, too!)

Traditional breakfast foods don't always have to be served. Last night's leftovers or a peanut butter sandwich can be offered, too. Your main concern should be that your child eats something nutritious to give her the best start on the day. Breakfast is important because it provides her a significant amount of nutrients. If she misses breakfast, it will be difficult for her to compensate for this loss of nutrition later. Breakfast is a habit you want her to have and keep throughout her life.

What's the Best Way to Teach Table Manners?

Table manners are established over time, but again, they're a reflection of parents. Being a good act to follow will help your child establish behavioral guidelines for himself.

When possible, especially at the family dinner, set the table. Even if you use informal dinnerware or paper plates, or are eating a pizza, make setting the table a habit. By doing so, you'll feel better about serving your meals—especially ones that take time to prepare—and your child will grow up with a sense of proper table etiquette. This habit will also make your child feel secure and comfortable in other eating situations.

And don't forget that children need to be comfortable while they eat. How would you like to sit at a table that's chin-high? When a chair is too large or your child's feet dangle and have no place to rest, he'll become irritable quickly. Children need to be comfortable, just as adults, in order to enjoy their meals. Booster seats, telephone books, or blocks to rest feet on can help balance a child and make him comfortable during a meal.

Set rules and be consistent but not too rigid. Remember that the attention span of a toddler is only 15 to 20 minutes, so excuse your little one from the table if he is finished eating. Older children should be able to sit through 20 to 30 minute meals.

Children as young as 1 to 2 years begin using small utensils to feed themselves, but they don't master feeding skills until they are 4 or 5. A 4-year-old should be able to comfortably use a fork, spoon, and knife (for spreading), napkin, drink solely from a small unbreakable glass, and use language such as "please," "thank you," and "excuse me." Using a knife for cutting isn't usually mastered until a child is 6 to 8 years old.

Messes and spills are a part of every toddler's life so your little one should not be reprimanded while she's learning. If you're really concerned about messes, try using plastic dinnerware, plates with separate compartments (to help keep food from getting mixed together), floor mats, and bibs. (Tarps in the kitchen are probably overdoing it, however.)

Some mealtime behaviors, such as throwing food and purposely spilling beverages, are inappropriate at any age and should be stopped immediately. As previously mentioned, when your child exhibits this type of behavior, simply remove him from the table and remind him that this is not acceptable behavior. Rewarding him with food for being good, or taking foods away when he is bad, should not become a habit. Behavior problems could become an everyday occurrence for attention and lead to a lifetime of problems.

Mealtimes should be an enjoyable time for everyone. Take a flexible, relaxed approach to eating. When the family enjoys food and each other, mealtime is more pleasant for everyone and children grow up with positive self-esteem.

Chapter 10

Answers to the Most Commonly Asked Questions from Parents of Young Children

Is my child getting the right foods?

If we wanted to split hairs, it's not the right foods that are important, it's the right *nutrients* and in the right quantities. But of
course, we need to eat the right foods to get the right nutrients.

Everyone needs the same nutrients, but in varying amounts.
Children need an abundance of nutrients, but they don't need to
eat as much as adults. Children should eat at least five servings of
fruits and vegetables, and two servings of protein-rich foods
(meat, eggs, and beans) daily. But the serving sizes are adjusted as
your child grows. A 2-year-old needs 2 tablespoons of vegetables
and a 4-year-old needs 4 tablespoons or 1/4 cup as a serving. At

least three to four servings of milk or milk products and a minimum of six servings of breads and cereals should all be included in daily meal planning to meet the nutrients needs of growing children. Refer to pages 41 and 52 for more information.

Are junk foods bad for my child?

There are no good and bad foods, therefore *no* food needs to be totally eliminated from the diet. High-fat, high-sugar, empty-calorie foods, most commonly known as "junk foods" (candy, cookies, chips, soft drinks, desserts, and fatty foods), are not bad for your child on occasion. It's the daily eating of these foods that should be avoided. These foods are labeled unhealthy or junk foods because they contribute no significant amount of nutrition. Since your child's overall physical capacity is small and she needs healthful foods to grow, her diet should consist of the foods outlined in the Food Guide Pyramid, with an occasional treat. Too many sweets, high-fat snacks, and less healthful choices could become a problem. Refer to pages 41 and 43 for more information.

Are artificially sweetened foods harmful to my child?

You may prefer foods sweetened with artificial and non-nutritive sweeteners, but they're not the best foods for your child. Children need calories and nutrients from a variety of foods to grow and develop. If your child fills up on artificial or non-nutritive sweeteners that do not contain all the nutrients he needs, he may not have room for foods that do. An occasional artificially sweetened product won't hurt, but it should not become a habit. Refer to page 68 for more information.

Does my child need a vitamin/mineral supplement?

Eating foods from all the major food groups will supply your child with enough vitamins and minerals necessary for growth. By encouraging your child to eat a variety of foods you will lead her to a lifetime of good eating habits. If you don't think she's getting enough vitamins and minerals, talk to your doctor. A daily, chewable multivitamin with no more than 100 percent of the RDA (Recommended Dietary Allowance) for children will not harm your child, but it's probably not necessary. If multivitamins are in your home, be sure they're sealed with a child-proof lid and kept in a medicine cabinet away from children. Your child may be harmed if she has more than one a day. Multivitamin supplements sometimes come in fun shapes, but children need to know that vitamins are not candy. Refer to page 71 for more information.

How do I know if my child is eating enough?

Children's appetites are unpredictable and varied. Their meal patterns may be so erratic that it's difficult to determine if they're eating enough. Recording your child's height and weight can be a good way to reassure yourself. If he's gaining weight and growing taller, there's no reason to be concerned about his eating patterns. Discuss your concerns with your doctor. Remember that preschool children only need 1,000 to 1,500 calories each day. That's about half the quantity adults need. So don't compare the quantity of what you eat with that of your child. Just make sure you offer him healthy foods to meet his daily calorie requirements. Refer to page 40 for more information.

What should I do if my child would rather snack throughout the day than sit down and eat a meal?

Stop and think why she might not want to sit down and eat. Are meals and snacks separated by at least 1 and 1/2 to 2 hours? Are mealtimes pleasant with conversation in which she can take part? Does the rest of the family sit down together and eat? Is meal-time TV time instead of family time? Are you asking her to sit in place for longer than 15 or 20 minutes? Is she comfortable at the table?

Meals need to be scheduled at approximately the same time each day. Children like schedules. It's difficult for a child who is accustomed to eating around 5:30 p.m. to suddenly wait until 7:00 p.m. Your child should be given a beginning and ending to snacks, as well as meals. This eliminates "nibbling" throughout the day. Keep in mind that the more pleasurable mealtime is made, the more she'll want to enjoy it with the family. Refer to pages 48 and 98 for more information.

What are easy-to-prepare sources of protein, other than cheese and peanut butter?

Preschoolers only need a small amount of protein each day, the amount you find in about 2 to 3 ounces of meat. While protein is important, children don't need a lot of it. Other good sources of protein include eggs, cottage cheese, yogurt, sliced turkey, chicken, and beef, tuna, and foods made with milk such as soups or even pudding. Refer to page 86 for more information.

What should I do about my child who wants the same food day after day?

Children's food jags (eating only one or two foods day after day) have always caused problems for parents. The first step is to relax and realize this is both normal and temporary. A few weeks may seem long to you, but in the growth of a child, it's not. Don't call attention to his behavior. Continue to serve your regular meal, and do not force your child to eat what you are having. Generally, when children see parents are not upset and refuse to give attention to this behavior, the children will become more accepting of other foods. Common food jags are peanut butter sandwiches, pizza, macaroni and cheese, and dry cereal with milk. These foods all make big contributions to a healthy diet. Refer to page 43 for more information.

Should I force my child to eat if she's not interested?

Forcing her to eat will cause dinnertime behavior problems, and will not result in nourishing her. She should be encouraged to try all the foods offered. Set good examples by serving the same foods to every family member and eating these foods yourself. Do not reinforce negative behavior by giving it too much attention. Refer to page 44 for more information.

How can I get my child to eat vegetables?

One way to introduce your family, especially your child to different vegetables, is to choose a different one frequently and ask your child to help you prepare it. Offer a wide variety of vegetables prepared in different ways, both cooked and raw with a dip. Encourage him to at least try a bite. Talking about the vegetable—where and how it's grown, its color, and so forth—may interest him to the point of experimenting with taste. More importantly, let your child form his own opinions. If you or another family member announces, "I don't like green vegetables," your child may decide against them, too. It's important to be a good role model. Refer to page 87 for more information.

Should I worry about cholesterol?

Parents should be concerned about cholesterol in their child's diet IF the family has a history of heart disease (family members under the age of 60 who have had heart attacks or strokes). Children of parents with high cholesterol levels are more likely to have high levels compared with other children.

At-risk children should have their blood cholesterol levels measured after the age of 2 years. Consult your doctor. Children at risk need to change their eating habits and have an active lifestyle to best prevent heart disease. Create more games and activities that involve exercising and less television and sitting. Refer to page 66 for more information.

What should I do if my child does not like milk?

Milk is a major source of calcium and also provides significant amounts of protein, vitamins A and D, and riboflavin. If your child does not like milk, try dairy products like yogurt, cheese, cottage cheese, or flavored milks (chocolate, strawberry, banana) and instant breakfast drinks. Also, add milk or non-fat dry milk powder to hot cereals, scrambled eggs, macaroni and cheese, soups, or other recipes to boost their calcium content. Continue to offer your child milk at regular intervals remembering that her food habits may change—they're not set in stone at this age. Refer to page 89 for more information.

When can my child start to drink skim milk?

Doctors and registered dietitians do not recommend skim milk for children under 2. Prior to this time, children need the additional calories provided by the fat in whole milk. A more appropriate choice after age 2 may be switching to low-fat or 2 percent milk, which contains less fat than whole milk, but has a heavier consistency than skim milk. Refer to page 27 for more information.

How can I get my child to try new foods?

One of the best ways to get a child to try new foods is to be a good role model. You need to eat the foods that you'd like your child to try. If he sees you eating something new, he's more likely to try it (although this might not happen immediately). Remember to serve the new food first during the meal when your child is the most hungry. Another suggestion is to let him help with the food preparation to spur his interest in the food. Refer to page 47 for more information.

What are some creative, nutritious food ideas?

Let your child pick a theme meal, such as Mexican, Chinese, or Mickey Mouse. She can then help decide what foods, plates, and garnishes to use. Work with her to plan a well-balanced meal including all groups from the Food Pyramid. She can also be creative with utensils, cookie cutters, and popsicle sticks to make various sandwich shapes or kabobs. Using small fresh fruits and vegetables such as cherry tomatoes, olives, raisins, and grapes to decorate foods add a special touch. Refer to page 91 for more information.

When is the best time to introduce baby foods?

Solid foods (baby foods) are usually introduced between the age of 4 to 6 months when your baby can sit up, accept a spoon, and swallow solid food easily. First foods should be a supplement to breast milk or formula, not a replacement. Iron fortified rice cereal is usually the first solid food introduced because it is non-allergenic and tolerated by most infants.

Cereals and other solid foods should always be fed by spoon. Never put cereal in the bottle or a syringe-type feeder. Offer food in small quantities of 1 to 2 tablespoons until your baby becomes accustomed to the food and spoon. Be patient and allow yourself extra time for meals. This should be an enjoyable experience for both parent and baby. Refer to page 27 for more information.

Is it safe to reuse baby food from jars?

If your baby cannot eat an entire jar of baby food, spoon half onto a plate and refrigerate the rest. Heat only the portion you plan to use at one time and discard any leftovers on the plate. If you feed your baby straight from the jar and he cannot finish it, throw the remainder away. By moving the spoon between the baby's mouth and the food, his saliva is added to the food in the jar, making the food thin and watery. In this state, it's not appropriate to refrigerate the food and use it again. Refer to page 32 for more information.

Can I reuse a bottle if my baby doesn't finish all of it from an earlier feeding?

Formula is a perfect food in which bacteria grows. It's nourishing and warm. Through trial and error, you'll realize the amount of formula your baby will drink at each feeding, resulting in less leftovers. Once a bottle has been warmed for feeding (or even if it's prepared to feed at room temperature), any unused formula should not be refrigerated—it should be thrown away. Refer to page 24 for more information.

How can I get my child to drink milk instead of juice during meal and snack time?

Set rules for meals and snacks, and be consistent. Try alternating milk then juice at meals and snacks, or set a rule in which only milk will be consumed at meals and juice or milk at snacks. Sometimes when your child is thirsty, offer water. It's a better thirst quencher than juice or milk.

What are some positive ways to encourage healthy eating?

Start by serving healthful foods at meals, as well as at snack time. If you eat healthful foods, you'll encourage your child to do the same. Try the following ideas and refer to page 87 for more information:

- modify family meals to appeal to small children
- provide an enjoyable mealtime environment
- don't insist that your child "clean the plate"
- serve child-sized portions
- don't offer food as a bribe, reward, or comfort
- limit "convenience" foods that are high in fat, sugar, and sodium
- concentrate on the nutrition your child is getting, rather than how much he is eating
- make snacks as nutritious as the food served at meals

What are some healthy, fast, and easy snacks?

Many children tend to snack on the same foods day after day because their parents choose prepackaged convenience foods. However, there are many alternatives to the all-too-common cookies and snack crackers. Refer to page 48 for more information. A few alternatives are listed below:

- graham crackers
- mini rice cakes
- breadsticks
- oatmeal-raisin cookies
- grapes
- apple/pear/orange sections
- cheddar cheese cubes
- juice popsicles
- carrot/celery sticks
- mini-bagels
- pretzels, hard and soft
- gingersnaps/vanilla wafers
- raisins
- cantaloupe/watermelon balls
- yogurt raisins
- mozzarella cheese sticks
- dried fruit
- cucumber slices

What should I do if my child won't eat fruits or vegetables?

More than likely this is a temporary phase. Children who avoid fruits and vegetables are most likely eating large amounts of other foods, which are probably high in fat, sugar, and calories. In other words, your child may be loading up on cookies, chips, candy bars, or dessert cakes—even meats and breads—instead of fruits and vegetables, which provide more vitamins, minerals, fiber, and less calories.

It's important for children to eat fruits and vegetables because many adult diseases like cancer, heart disease, diabetes, and obesity are more commonly found in societies where people do not regularly eat fruits and vegetables. Try incorporating fruit and vegetable juices into your child's diet. And look for interesting fresh fruits and vegetables at the supermarket that may appeal to you and your child. Refer to page 89 for more information.

If my child refuses foods at dinner, should I make him something else?

Children have strong likes and dislikes, but they do not need to be served different foods than the family at meals. Although it's a good idea to keep your child's favorites in mind, it's easiest and most sensible to make only one meal for the family. Let your child choose the foods from the meal he would like to eat, but don't insist or force him to eat anything else. Your child needs to be exposed to a variety of foods, but when you're offering a new food, try to also include one that is familiar and something he likes. Children will be more likely to try new foods and enjoy family meals if they are comfortable with the foods presented to them. Refer to page 45 for more information.

What should I do if my child won't eat meals or misses a meal entirely?

The less attention you pay to a missed meal the better. Don't reward your child with foods you wouldn't feed at mealtime. Wait until your child announces that she is hungry and reoffer the missed meal or some appropriate nutritional equivalent. Refer to page 56 for more information.

When should I expect my child to behave at the table?

By age 1, children can understand what behavior will not be tolerated at the table. Children should learn their basic table manners by watching other family members. Set reasonable rules for your child's age and be consistent. Being too strict on your child may frustrate him and make things worse. From younger children expect some spills and messes to be true accidents, not deliberate. Older children should be expected to sit through a meal, but toddlers should be excused early if necessary. Try to keep table conversation pleasant and put less emphasis on what and how much your child is eating. Also, remember that your child likes to please you, so be sure to praise him for desirable behavior. Refer to pages 34 and 99 for more information.

Where to Go for More Information

American Academy of Pediatrics

141 Northwest Pt. Blvd.
Elk Grove Village, IL 60007-1098
Has public education material available on children's health and nutrition.

American Dietetic Association
National Center for Nutrition and Dietetics

216 W. Jackson Blvd
Chicago, IL 60604
(consumer hotline: 800-366-1655)
Offers materials on nutrition. Registered dietitians are available for questions or to refer people to local professionals.

American Heart Association

7320 Greenville Ave.
Dallas, TX 75231
(214) 373-6300
Offers publications, fact sheets, and brochures on topics related to heart disease risk prevention, exercise, and nutrition.

Consumer Information Center

Pueblo, CO 81009
Provides free or low-cost consumer booklets on such topics as nutrition, exercise, smoking, etc.

Food and Drug Administration

Office of Consumer Affairs
5600 Fishers Lane
Rockville, MD 20857
(301) 443-3170
Has information available on developments in the areas of food safety and regulations, drugs, pesticides, and cosmetics.

La Leche League International

9616 Minneapolis Ave., P.O. Box 1209
Franklin Park, IL 60131-8209
(800) LA LECHE or (800) 525-3243
Provides encouragement and support to nursing mothers and breast feeding resource materials.

National Dairy Council

6300 N. River Rd.
Rosemont, IL 60018
(800) 426-8271
Offers guides to good eating and nutrition during pregnancy and childhood. Can also refer people to their local affiliates.

U.S. Department of Agriculture

Food and Nutrition Information Center
National Agricultural Library
10301 Baltimore Blvd.
Beltsville, MD 20705
(301) 504-5917
Offers food and nutrition database searches and information on resource guides and preschool child nutrition programs.

What Counts as a Serving?

	Pregnancy/ Lactating	Toddler	Preschooler
Breads, Cereals, Rice, and Pasta			
Bread	1 slice	1/4-1/2 slice	1/2 slice
Cooked rice or pasta	1/2 cup	1/4 cup	1/3 cup
Cooked cereal	1/2 cup	1/4 cup	1/3 cup
Ready-to-eat cereal	1 ounce	1/4 cup	1/3 cup
Vegetables			
Cooked	1/2 cup	2 tbsp.	1/4 cup
Raw	1/2-1 cup	2 tbsp.	1/4 cup
Fruits			
Fresh fruit	1 piece	2 tbsp.	1/4 cup
Juice	3/4 cup	1/4 cup	1/2 cup
Canned fruit	1/2 cup	1/4 cup	1/2 cup
Milk, Yogurt, Cheese			
Milk or yogurt	1 cup	1/2 cup	3/4 cup
Cheese	1 1/2-2 ounces	1 ounce	1 1/2 ounce
Meat, Poultry, Fish, Dry Beans, Eggs, Nuts			
Lean meat	1 1/2 -3 ounces	1 ounce	1 1/2 ounces
Cooked beans	1/2 cup*	2 tbsp.	1/4 cup
Egg	1*	1/2	1
Peanut Butter	2 tbsp.*	1 tbsp.	2 tbsp.

*Count as 1 ounce of meat or 1/3 serving.

Food Guide Pyramid

A Guide to Daily Food Choices

Suggested Minimum Servings Per Day

Fats, Oils, & Sweets
Use sparingly

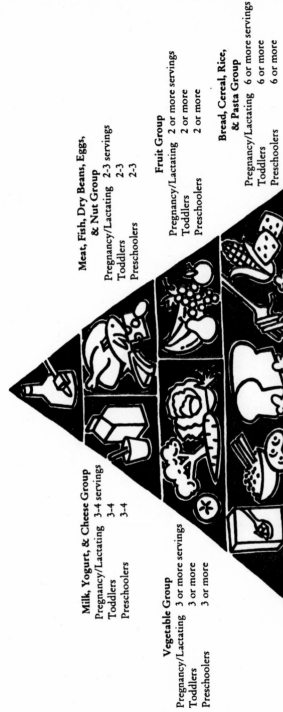

Milk, Yogurt, & Cheese Group

Pregnancy/Lactating	3-4 servings
Toddlers	3-4
Preschoolers	3-4

Vegetable Group

Pregnancy/Lactating	3 or more servings
Toddlers	3 or more
Preschoolers	3 or more

Meat, Fish, Dry Beans, Eggs, & Nut Group

Pregnancy/Lactating	2-3 servings
Toddlers	2-3
Preschoolers	2-3

Fruit Group

Pregnancy/Lactating	2 or more servings
Toddlers	2 or more
Preschoolers	2 or more

Bread, Cereal, Rice, & Pasta Group

Pregnancy/Lactating	6 or more servings
Toddlers	6 or more
Preschoolers	6 or more

Illustration: Jan Westberg

115

RECIPES

Initially, we hadn't planned to include recipes in this book. However, we quickly changed our minds after asking parents of young children what advice or tools they needed to feed their children nutritiously and appropriately. One subject that continually came up was, "Where can I get healthy, fun, and nutritious recipes that will satisfy my child, be easy to prepare, and be appropriate for my whole family as well?"

That's quite a request. (Some would say a difficult if not impossible request!) But we were up to the task.

Here we provide over 50 of our favorite recipes that are quick, easy, and nutritious at the same time. Plus, they're foods that can be enjoyed by everyone and a great start to a family recipe file.

Get children involved in meal and snack preparation at an early age. Begin with menu planning, shopping for ingredients, measuring, pouring, mixing, and watching the finished product take shape—then, best of all, enjoying the foods together. There's no better way to teach your young child about food and get him off to a good, nutritional start.

When analyzing these recipes, the following decisions were made:

- Nutritional information is indicated for calories, protein, carbohydrates, and fat. Figures are rounded off to the closest whole number. The recipes are analyzed using The Food Processor II Software, ESHA Research, Salem, OR and Nutritionist III, N-Squared Computing, Salem, OR.

- Portion sizes are indicated for children and may not be the appropriate size for adults.

- Ingredients listed as optional are not included in the nutrient analysis.

- Milk included in recipes is analyzed as 2 percent milk.

- When no specific type of flour or sugar is indicated, standard-white was used.

- When beef is used in recipes, we allow for meat to be lean and free of excess fat.

- Because most children do not need to restrict their fat intake if they have a balanced diet, light or unrestricted fat products were not used in preparing recipes. Occasional substitutions of these products in recipes (i.e. light cream cheese, light sour cream, light mayonnaise) are not harmful, but should not be used exclusively.

Notes: For young children (under age 2) use whole milk for recipes calling for milk because fat should not be restricted in their diets. To increase fiber and nutrition in recipes, substitute brown rice for white rice, whole-wheat flour for white flour, and add wheat germ, granola, or rolled oats when possible.

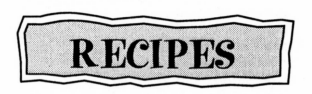

RECIPES

Soups
Easy Chicken Soup
Veggie Chowder
Creamy Potato Soup

Main Courses
Oven Baked Drumsticks
Chicken Fajitas
Your Own Baked Chicken Nuggets
Baked Chicken with Noodles
Skilletburgers
Hamburger Veggie Casserole
Family Meat Loaf
Teriyaki Meatballs
Easy Baked Fish
Baked Tuna Balls
Children's Favorite Salmon Patties
Vegetable Pizza Pocket
Easy Macaroni and Cheese
Creative Peanut Butter Sandwiches

Vegetables
Tasty Spinach Casserole
Baked Carrots with Raisins
Quick and Easy Fried Rice
Fruited Rice
Vegetable Dip
Bite Sized Potato Skins
Baked Parmesan Potato Fries
Apple Cinnamon Couscous

Salads

Tortellini Cheese Salad
Yum Yum Salad
Ice Cream Salad
Fresh Fruit Salad
Lemonade Cheese Mold

Breads

Chocolate Chip Banana Bread
Oatmeal Buttermilk Pancakes
Applesauce Breakfast Cake
Pumpkin Cream Cheese Muffins
Oatmeal Muffins
Watch 'em Grow Popovers
Cinnamon Cream Cheese Bites

Desserts

Lemon Zucchini Cookies
Spice Squares
Low-fat Lemon Squares
Oatmeal Raisin Cookies
Carrot Brownies
Bread Pudding
Chocolate Peanutty Banana Lollipops
Orange Fruit Pie
Rainbow Fruit Kabobs
Frozen Rainbow Sandwiches
Orange Yogurt Popsicles
Baked Apple Cobbler
Apple Cheese Crisp

Beverages

Sherbetty Fruit Punch
Yogurt Strawberry Smoothie

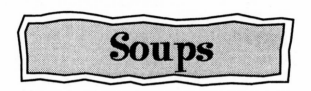

Easy Chicken Soup

The entire family will enjoy this easy-to-make chicken soup. Try variations with different vegetables or add cooked pasta. Children love it with alphabet noodles.

Servings: 16

Ingredients:

3 pounds chicken, cut up
3 carrots, cut up
3 celery stalks, cut up
2 onions, cut up
salt and pepper as desired

Method:

Rinse chicken under cold water.

Place chicken with remaining ingredients in 4 quarts of cold water. Bring to a boil.

Cover and simmer for approximately 3 hours until chicken is tender and falls off bones easily.

Each serving contains:

Calories: 54
Protein: 5 grams
Carbohydrates: 4 grams
Fat: 1 gram

Veggie Chowder

Use whatever vegetable leftovers you have to create different versions of this chowder. It's a meal in itself!

Servings: 6

Ingredients:

2 cups water
1 10 3/4-ounce can chicken broth
1 cup sliced carrots
1/2 cup chopped onions
1 clove minced garlic
1 cup chopped fresh broccoli
1 cup chopped cauliflower
2 tablespoons flour
3/4 cup milk
1 1/2 cups shredded Swiss cheese
salt and pepper to taste

Method:

In large saucepan, combine water, broth, carrots, onion, and garlic. Bring to boil. Add broccoli and cauliflower. Return mixture to boiling.

Cover and simmer for 8 to 10 minutes.

Stir flour into milk until smooth. Add slowly to boiling soup. Cook until soup thickens, about 10 minutes.

Just before serving, stir cheese into soup.

Each serving contains:

Calories: 168
Protein: 12 grams
Carbohydrates: 11 grams
Fat: 9 grams

Creamy Potato Soup

A nice accompaniment to salad, a half sandwich, or by itself, this soup is especially good on a cold, winter day.

Servings: 10

Ingredients:

4 tablespoons margarine
1 cup chopped onion
4 cups peeled & chopped potatoes
1 chopped carrot
2 cups water
1 teaspoon dill
3 cups milk
2 tablespoons parsley
salt and pepper to taste

Method:

In large saucepan, saute onion in margarine. Add potatoes, carrot, water, and dill. Bring to a boil.
Cover and simmer until potatoes are tender, approximately 20 to 30 minutes.
Add milk and parsley. Return to boiling.

Each serving contains:

Calories: 144
Protein: 4 grams
Carbohydrates: 19 grams
Fat: 6 grams

Main Courses

Oven Baked Drumsticks

Most children love chicken drumsticks. These drumsticks are easy, and best of all, they're not fried.

Servings: 6

Ingredients:

1/2 cup flour
1 teaspoon salt
1/2 teaspoon paprika
1/4 teaspoon pepper
1/4 cup melted margarine
6 chicken drumsticks

Method:

Preheat oven to 425 degrees.
Mix flour, salt, paprika, and pepper in small bowl.
Coat drumsticks in melted margarine and roll in flour mixture.
Set drumsticks on ungreased pan or cookie sheet.
Bake about 50 minutes or until fully cooked.

Each serving contains:

Calories: 224
Protein: 15 grams
Carbohydrates: 8 grams
Fat: 14 grams

Chicken Fajitas

Children love rolling foods in tortillas. Chicken is a favorite, but beef and cheese work well, too.

Servings: 6

Ingredients:

3 boneless, skinless chicken breasts
2 teaspoons soy sauce
1/4 cup lime juice
3 cloves garlic, minced
1/2 cup chopped onion
1/2 cup chopped green pepper
1 tomato, chopped
6 flour tortillas

Method:

Mix soy sauce, lime juice, and garlic together. Marinate chicken in mixture for at least 1 hour.
Grill or broil chicken. Cool slightly. Slice into thin strips.
Chop vegetables into small pieces. (Vegetables can either be raw or slightly sauteed.)
Roll chicken strips and vegetables in tortilla. Serve warm.

Each serving contains:

Calories: 185
Protein: 17 grams
Carbohydrates: 23 grams
Fat: 4 grams

Your Own Baked Chicken Nuggets

It's always nice to have chicken bites handy for a quick meal. Try making your own. They're fast, easy, and best of all, not fried.

Servings: 6

Ingredients:

3 boneless, skinless chicken breasts
2 tablespoons flour
1/4 teaspoon salt
1/4 teaspoon pepper
2 tablespoons milk
3/4 cup bread crumbs

Method:

Preheat oven to 425 degrees.
Cut chicken into bite-sized pieces.
Combine flour, salt, and pepper in small bowl. Place milk in another small bowl. In yet another small bowl, place bread crumbs.
Dip chicken in flour mixture, then in milk, and finally in bread crumbs. Place on cookie sheet.
Bake 15 minutes until golden brown and cooked throughout.

Each serving contains:

Calories: 132
Protein: 15 grams
Carbohydrates: 11 grams
Fat: 2 grams

Baked Chicken with Noodles

This all-in-one dish is one your whole family is sure to enjoy. It also makes a great leftover treat the next day.

Servings: 6

Ingredients:

2 cups cooked, diced, chicken breast
1 10 3/4-ounce can cream of chicken soup
1/2 cup milk
2 tablespoons diced pimento
1 tablespoon chopped parsley
2 cups cooked noodles
1/4 cup bread crumbs

Method:

Preheat oven to 350 degrees.
Blend soup and milk. Add chicken, pimento, parsley, and noodles.
Spoon into casserole dish. Sprinkle with bread crumbs.
Bake 25 to 30 minutes.

Each serving contains:

Calories: 192
Protein: 13 grams
Carbohydrates: 21 grams
Fat: 5 grams

Skilletburgers

This quick and easy meal only requires one pan, so clean up is a breeze. It's delicious served on a toasted bun or even over a bed of rice.

Servings: 8

Ingredients:

1 1/4 pounds ground beef
1 large onion, chopped
1 medium green pepper, chopped
1/2 teaspoon salt
2/3 cup catsup
2 tablespoons sugar
2 tablespoons mustard
1 tablespoon vinegar

Method:

Brown ground beef in skillet. Drain fat. Add chopped onion and pepper and saute.
Add remaining ingredients to beef mixture. Simmer 30 minutes.

Each serving contains:

Calories: 241
Protein: 18 grams
Carbohydrates: 11 grams
Fat: 14 grams

Hamburger Veggie Casserole

Meat, vegetables, and pasta together make this a one-dish meal.
Servings: 8

Ingredients:

1 pound ground beef
1/2 cup chopped onion
1 tablespoon vegetable oil
1/2 teaspoon salt
1 16-ounce can mixed vegetables
2 cups cooked macaroni
3 tablespoons catsup
pepper, as desired

Method:

Brown ground beef and onion in oil. Drain excess fat.
Add remaining ingredients. Simmer until most of the liquid has cooked out.

Each serving contains:

Calories: 243
Protein: 17 grams
Carbohydrates: 15 grams
Fat: 13 grams

Family Meat Loaf

Here's a family favorite. It can also be made in a cupcake pan for individual portions—served with a scoop of mashed potatoes with a cherry tomato on top. What a fun meal!

Servings: 12

Ingredients:

1 tablespoon vegetable oil
1 cup chopped onion
1/2 cup celery, chopped
1 minced garlic clove
1/4 cup milk
1/4 cup seasoned bread crumbs
1 1/2 pounds ground beef

2 eggs
2 tablespoons Parmesan cheese
1 tablespoon Worcestershire
   sauce
1 tablespoon parsley
1/4 teaspoon pepper

Method:

Preheat oven to 375 degrees.
Heat oil in skillet. Saute onion, celery, and garlic until onion is tender, 4 to 5 minutes.
In large bowl, combine milk and bread crumbs, until bread crumbs are softened, about 3 minutes.
Add remaining ingredients to bread crumb mixture, including onion and celery.
Turn mixture into meat loaf pan. Bake 1 hour.
Cool slightly before slicing.

Each serving contains:

Calories: 200
Protein: 16 grams
Carbohydrates: 4 grams
Fat: 13 grams

Teriyaki Meatballs

These delicious meatballs can be served on popsicle sticks. Just watch them go as if they're lollipops.

Servings: 12 (24 meatballs)

Ingredients:

1 scallion, chopped
6 tablespoons teriyaki sauce
3 tablespoons catsup
1 egg
1/4 cup bread crumbs
1 pound ground beef

Method:

Preheat oven to 400 degrees.
Combine scallion, 2 tablespoons of teriyaki sauce, 1 tablespoon of catsup, the egg, bread crumbs, and beef in a large bowl.
Shape mixture into approximately 24 balls. Place into baking dish.
Combine remaining teriyaki sauce and catsup. Brush mixture on top of meatballs.
Bake about 15 minutes. Turn meatballs. Bake additional 10 to 15 minutes.

Each serving contains:

Calories: 129
Protein: 11 grams
Carbohydrates: 4 grams
Fat: 8 grams

Easy Baked Fish

Nutritious, quick, and easy, too. Children enjoy eating fish. Try to serve fish more often.

Servings: 6

Ingredients:

1 pound fillet of sole or white fish fillets
2 teaspoons lemon juice
1/2 cup seasoned bread crumbs
1/8 teaspoon salt
1/8 teaspoon pepper
1 tablespoon parsley flakes
2 tablespoons margarine

Method:

Place fish in baking dish and sprinkle with lemon juice and bread crumbs. Season with salt, pepper, and parsley. Dot fish with cut up margarine.

Bake at 400 degrees for approximately 15 minutes until fish is golden brown and flakes easily with a fork when pricked.

Garnish with fresh lemon slices.

Each serving contains:

Calories: 150
Protein: 16 grams
Carbohydrates: 9 grams
Fat: 5 grams

Baked Tuna Balls

These can be served with a fork or eaten as finger food, dipped in tartar sauce. For variety, try adding cheese before cooking. Children love them.

Servings: 12 (approximately 24 balls)

Ingredients:

2 6 1/2-ounce cans water packed tuna, drained and flaked
1 1/2 cups cornflake crumbs
1/3 cup mayonnaise
1 egg
1 teaspoon minced onion
1 teaspoon mustard

Method:

Preheat oven to 400 degrees.
Combine tuna, 1 cup of the cornflake crumbs, mayonnaise, egg, onion, and mustard.
Shape mixture into balls approximately 1-inch in diameter.
Roll balls in remaining cornflake crumbs and place on baking dish.
Bake for approximately 20 minutes, until golden brown.

Each serving contains:

Calories: 156
Protein: 12 grams
Carbohydrates: 14 grams
Fat: 6 grams

Children's Favorite Salmon Patties

A baked version of an old favorite. You can prepare these as indicated or experiment with various types of cheese. Every batch turns out delicious.

Servings: 6

Ingredients:

2 6 1/2-ounce cans, boneless, skinless salmon
1/2 cup seasoned bread crumbs
1 egg
1/4 cup shredded mozzarella cheese
1/2 teaspoon garlic powder

Method:

Preheat oven to 425 degrees.
Drain salmon, reserving 2 teaspoons liquid. Combine liquid from salmon and all ingredients in bowl.
Shape in 4 to 6 patties.
Bake approximately 20 minutes until patties are golden brown.
Serve with tartar sauce.

Each serving contains:

Calories: 169
Protein: 17 grams
Carbohydrates: 10 grams
Fat: 6 grams

Vegetable Pizza Pocket

A great lunch idea that your child can help prepare. And the options for variations with different types of vegetables are endless.

Servings: 2

Ingredients:

1 large pita bread circle
1/4 cup spaghetti sauce
1/4 cup shredded mozzarella cheese
2 tablespoons chopped green pepper
2 tablespoons chopped onion
1/4 teaspoon garlic powder

Method:

Cut pita bread circle in half. Open each half carefully.
Insert half of the ingredients in each pocket.
Place pockets on microwaveable plate and microwave approximately 2 minutes until cheese is melted.
Cool slightly before serving.

Each serving contains:

Calories: 201
Protein: 11 grams
Carbohydrates: 23 grams
Fat: 7 grams

Easy Macaroni and Cheese

A staple for many families—it's easier and more nutritious to prepare from scratch rather than from a box.

Servings: 8

Ingredients:

8 ounces macaroni noodles
2 tablespoons melted margarine
1 cup milk
8 ounces shredded cheddar cheese

Method:

Preheat oven to 350 degrees.
Prepare macaroni according to package directions. Drain.
Combine remaining ingredients in 2-quart baking dish.
Add macaroni.
Bake for 35 to 45 minutes until bubbly.

Each serving contains:

Calories: 259
Protein: 12 grams
Carbohydrates: 23 grams
Fat: 13 grams

Creative Peanut Butter Sandwiches

If your child insists on peanut butter sandwiches daily, be creative. The options with these are endless. Let your child choose their shape and filling. Also, substitute graham crackers for bread for a real treat.

Servings: 4

Ingredients:

4 slices bread
1/4 cup peanut butter
2 tablespoons mashed banana (or try one of the following for
    variety: applesauce, diced apples, diced pineapple, grated carrots)

Method:

Use small cookie cutters to cut bread into desired shape or cut into small strips, squares, or triangles.
Combine peanut butter and banana. Spread onto bread. Assemble sandwiches.

Each serving contains:

Calories: 177
Protein: 7 grams
Carbohydrates: 18 grams
Fat: 9 grams

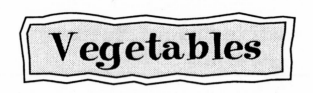

Vegetables

Tasty Spinach Casserole

You'd be surprised how children enjoy spinach when given the opportunity to try it. Tell them it's the food that makes Popeye so strong.

Servings: 8

Ingredients:

2 10-ounce packages chopped frozen spinach
4 ounces (1/2 of 8-ounce package) cream cheese
2 tablespoons melted margarine
1/4 teaspoon dry mustard
1/8 teaspoon paprika
dash nutmeg
salt and pepper, as desired

Method:

Preheat oven to 350 degrees.
Cook spinach according to package directions. Drain.
Add cream cheese and melted margarine to drained spinach.
Add dry mustard, paprika, nutmeg, salt, and pepper. Press into baking dish.
Bake until thoroughly heated through, about 15 to 20 minutes.

Each serving contains:

Calories: 95
Protein: 3 grams
Carbohydrates: 4 grams
Fat: 8 grams

Baked Carrots with Raisins

The raisins in this dish make it very attractive to young children. The color and taste attract their little appetites.

Servings: 8

Ingredients:

1 pound carrots, thinly sliced
1/4 cup raisins
1/4 cup margarine
3 tablespoons honey
1 tablespoon lemon juice
1/4 teaspoon ginger

Method:

Preheat oven to 375 degrees.
Cook carrots, covered, in 1/2 inch boiling water for 8 minutes. Drain.
Place carrots into baking dish. Add raisins, margarine, honey, lemon juice, and ginger.
Bake, uncovered, for 30 to 35 minutes, stirring occasionally.

Each serving contains:

Calories: 114
Protein: 1 gram
Carbohydrates: 16 grams
Fat: 6 grams

Quick and Easy Fried Rice

Fried rice is a family favorite because it goes with so many dishes. Variations to this recipe are unlimited. Try adding other vegetables (like broccoli, pea pods) or combine this with sliced or diced chicken for a meal-in-one.

Servings: 6

Ingredients:

1 1/2 cups uncooked instant rice
1/2 cup shredded carrot
1/4 cup chopped green onion
2 tablespoons soy sauce
1 tablespoon margarine
1/2 teaspoon garlic powder

Method:

Prepare rice according to package directions.
After rice is tender and water is absorbed, add remaining ingredients while fluffing with fork.

Each serving contains:

Calories: 115
Protein: 2 grams
Carbohydrates: 21 grams
Fat: 2 grams

Fruited Rice

This side dish adds color and taste to any meal. Your kids will love it and request it often.

Servings: 6

Ingredients:

1 10 1/2-ounce can condensed chicken broth
1 cup long grain rice
1/3 cup chopped green onion
2 tablespoons melted margarine
1 8 3/4-ounce can pineapple chunks, drained
2 tablespoons diced pimentos
1 tablespoon soy sauce

Method:

In saucepan, combine chicken broth and 1 soup can water. Bring to boil. Stir in rice and cover.
Simmer about 25 minutes, until liquid is absorbed.
Saute onion in margarine. Add pineapple and pimentos.
Heat thoroughly.
Combine cooked rice with pineapple mixture and soy sauce.

Each serving contains:

Calories: 189
Protein: 5 grams
Carbohydrates: 32 grams
Fat: 4 grams

Vegetable Dip

An easy-to-make dip for everyone to enjoy. Dip your favorite raw vegetables or try new ones, like squash, bell peppers, and cucumbers.

Servings: 10 (2 tablespoons per serving)

Ingredients:

1 cup cream style cottage cheese
1/4 cup buttermilk
1 teaspoon dried dill weed
pinch of salt

Method:

Mix all ingredients together in blender. Blend until smooth.

Each serving contains:

Calories: 12
Protein: 1 gram
Carbohydrates: 0 grams
Fat: 0 grams

Bite-Sized Potato Skins

A favorite among adults, children love these, too. Vary the recipe with other vegetables or allow your children to make their own.

Servings: 4

Ingredients:
1 large baked potato
1/4 cup plain low-fat yogurt
1/2 cup grated carrots (about 3 medium)
1/4 cup shredded cheddar cheese

Method:
Preheat oven to 350 degrees.

Cut cooked potato in half and scoop out inside (save for another dish), leaving skin intact. Cut skins in quarters, then in half again to make bite-sized pieces.

In small bowl, combine yogurt and carrots. Spoon yogurt mixture on each potato skin and top with cheese.

Bake approximately 10 minutes until cheese has melted. Cool before serving.

Each serving contains:
Calories: 72
Protein: 3 grams
Carbohydrates: 9 grams
Fat: 3 grams

Baked Parmesan Potato Fries

Try this version of a family staple. Crispy, tasty, but not too spicy.
Servings: 10

Ingredients:

1/2 cup bread crumbs
1/2 cup Parmesan cheese
1/8 teaspoon garlic powder
2 pounds potatoes
1 stick margarine, melted

Method:

Preheat oven to 400 degrees.
Combine bread crumbs, Parmesan cheese, and garlic powder.
Peel potatoes and cut lengthwise into thin strips.
Dip each strip in melted margarine and then coat with bread crumb mixture. Place on cookie sheet.
Bake 20 minutes. Turn. Bake an additional 20 minutes, until potatoes are tender and crispy.

Each serving contains:

Calories: 197
Protein: 4 grams
Carbohydrates: 22 grams
Fat: 11 grams

Apple Cinnamon Couscous

Growing in popularity, couscous (Moroccan pasta) is not only nutritious, but delicious. Try adding raisins to this dish for variety.

Servings: 6

Ingredients:

1 cup diced apple
1 tablespoon margarine
1 1/2 cups apple juice
1 teaspoon cinnamon
1 cup quick cooking couscous

Method:

In saucepan, combine all ingredients except couscous.
Bring to boil.
Add couscous, cover, and remove from heat.
Fluff with fork after 5 minutes.

Each serving contains:

Calories: 159
Protein: 3 grams
Carbohydrates: 31 grams
Fat: 2 grams

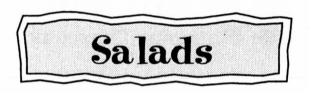

Salads

Tortellini Cheese Salad

This colorful dish is nutritious, delicious, and enjoyed by the whole family. It's great for guests, too.

Servings: 6

Ingredients:

6 ounces cheese-filled tortellini
1 cup mozzarella cheese, cubed
1/2 green pepper, thinly sliced
1/2 red pepper, thinly sliced
1/2 cup black olives, thinly sliced
1/2 cup Italian salad dressing
1/4 cup grated Parmesan cheese

Method:

Prepare tortellini according to package directions.
Drain tortellini when cooked and rinse with cold water.
Drain again.
Combine cheese, peppers, olives, and tortellini in large bowl. Toss with dressing. Sprinkle Parmesan cheese over salad before serving and toss lightly.

Each serving contains:

Calories: 299
Protein: 16 grams
Carbohydrates: 14 grams
Fat: 22 grams

Yum Yum Salad

Here's a salad your whole family will love. It's a delightful and colorful addition to any meal.

Servings: 12

Ingredients:

2 envelopes unflavored gelatin
1/2 cup cold water
1 20-ounce can crushed pineapple, drained
juice of 2 lemons
3/4 cup sugar
1/4 cup mayonnaise
1 cup shredded American cheese
1 cup heavy cream, lightly whipped

Method:

Dissolve gelatin in cold water.
In saucepan, heat pineapple, lemon juice, and sugar. Add to gelatin. Mix well. Chill until partially congealed.
Fold in mayonnaise, cheese, and cream. Pour into 9" x 9" pan. Chill until firm.
Cut into squares to serve.

Each serving contains:

Calories: 245
Protein: 6 grams
Carbohydrates: 19 grams
Fat: 17 grams

Ice Cream Salad

This delicious salad is great with a meal or as a dessert. Children can't resist it.

Servings: 6

Ingredients:

1 3-ounce package strawberry gelatin
1 cup boiling water
1 pint vanilla ice cream
1 16-ounce can fruit cocktail, drained

Method:

Dissolve gelatin in boiling water.
Add ice cream and stir until dissolved.
Add fruit cocktail. Pour into loaf pan. Chill until firm.

Each serving contains:

Calories: 169
Protein: 3 grams
Carbohydrates: 30 grams
Fat: 5 grams

Fresh Fruit Salad

A great summer treat. Guests and family alike always go for the fresh fruit when served in such a lovely manner.

Servings: 8

Ingredients:

2 peaches, sliced
1 cup blueberries
1 cup melon balls (cantaloupe or honeydew)
1 cup sliced strawberries
1 cup grapes
3 tablespoons orange juice
2/3 cup sour cream
3 tablespoons brown sugar

Method:

Toss fruit with orange juice.
Mix dressing of sour cream and brown sugar. Serve with fresh fruit.
Top fruit with sprinkle of brown sugar, if desired.

Each serving contains:

Calories: 117
Protein: 1 gram
Carbohydrates: 20 grams
Fat: 4 grams

Lemonade Cheese Mold

This colorful, delicious gelatin mold makes a nice side dish to any main course of meat, poultry, or fish. Let your little ones be creative by adding the strawberries and you'll see how impressed they'll be with the finished product.

Servings: 8

Ingredients:

1 envelope unflavored gelatin
1/4 cup cold water
1/2 cup boiling water
3 tablespoons sugar
6 ounces cream cheese
1 cup milk
1 6-ounce can frozen lemonade, thawed
1 cup sliced strawberries

Method:

Soften gelatin in cold water. Add boiling water and stir until completely dissolved.
Cream sugar into cream cheese. Slowly add milk.
Stir gelatin and lemonade into cream cheese mixture.
Pour into 1 quart ring mold. Refrigerate.
Serve with sliced strawberries.

Each serving contains:

Calories: 155
Protein: 3 grams
Carbohydrates: 18 grams
Fat: 8 grams

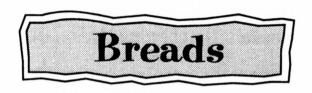

Chocolate Chip Banana Bread

Banana bread is a favorite among children. Adding chocolate chips makes it a real treat.

Servings: 2 loaves

Ingredients:

3/4 cup sugar
3 large mashed bananas
3/4 cup vegetable oil
2 eggs
2 cups flour
1 teaspoon baking soda
2 teaspoons vanilla
1/2 teaspoon baking powder
1/2 cup chocolate chips

Method:

Preheat oven to 325 degrees.
Grease two 9 x 5 x 3-inch loaf pans with vegetable spray.
Mix sugar, bananas, oil, and eggs into large bowl. Add remaining ingredients. Pour batter into pan. Fill 2/3 full.
Bake approximately 1 hour until toothpick inserted in center comes out clean. Cool completely before slicing.

Each serving contains:

Calories: 160
Protein: 2 grams
Carbohydrates: 20 grams
Fat: 9 grams

Oatmeal Buttermilk Pancakes

Here's a way to increase the nutritional content of an old favorite.
Servings: 12

Ingredients:

1/2 cup flour
1/2 cup quick cooking oats
3/4 cup buttermilk
1/4 cup milk
1 tablespoon sugar
2 tablespoons vegetable oil
1 teaspoon baking powder
1/2 teaspoon baking soda
1 egg
confectioners' sugar, as needed

Method:

Mix all ingredients until smooth.
Grease skillet as necessary.
When skillet is hot, pour approximately 1/4 cup batter on skillet.
Cook thoroughly until pancakes are puffy.
Turn and cook other side.
Sprinkle with confectioners' sugar before serving.

Each serving contains:

Calories: 71
Protein: 2 grams
Carbohydrates: 8 grams
Fat: 3 grams

Applesauce Breakfast Cake

Here's a nice alternative to a traditional breakfast. Your children will think it's a real treat eating cake for breakfast. Serve it warm or cold. It's great both ways.

Servings: 12

Topping:
1/4 cup brown sugar
1 tablespoon melted margarine
1/2 teaspoon cinnamon
1/4 cup chopped pecans

Cake:
1 cup flour
1/3 cup sugar
1/2 teaspoon baking powder
1/4 teaspoon baking soda
1 egg
1/2 cup applesauce
1/4 cup vegetable oil
1/2 teaspoon vanilla

Method:
Preheat oven to 350 degrees.
Spray 8-inch square baking pan with non-stick cooking spray.
In small bowl, mix brown sugar, margarine, and cinnamon until crumbly. Add chopped nuts.
In large bowl, mix together flour, sugar, baking powder, baking soda, and pinch of salt, if desired.
In another small bowl, beat egg slightly. Add applesauce, oil, and vanilla. Stir until mixed.
Add applesauce mixture to flour mixture. Stir until dry ingredients are wet. Pour batter into pan. Sprinkle topping over batter.
Bake 20 to 25 minutes. Cool.

Each serving contains:
Calories: 150
Protein: 2 grams
Carbohydrates: 19 grams
Fat: 8 grams

Pumpkin Cream Cheese Muffins

A delicious accompaniment to meals or in between as a snack.

Servings: 12

Ingredients:

2 eggs, lightly beaten
1/2 cup canned pumpkin
1/2 cup milk
1/4 cup vegetable oil
1 1/2 cups flour
1/3 cup sugar
1 tablespoon baking powder
1 teaspoon cinnamon
1/2 teaspoon nutmeg

Filling:

1 3-ounce package cream
  cheese, softened
1 tablespoon sugar
1 tablespoon milk

Method:

Preheat oven to 375 degrees.
Grease muffin tins.
Mix together eggs, pumpkin, milk, and oil. Add remaining ingredients.
Pour batter into muffin tins, 1/2 to 3/4 full.
Mix filling ingredients and top each muffin with 1 teaspoon.
Swirl filling into muffin batter with spatula or knife.
Bake approximately 20 minutes, until lightly browned. Cool.

Each serving contains:

Calories: 141
Protein: 3 grams
Carbohydrates: 19 grams
Fat: 6 grams

Oatmeal Muffins

These muffins are wonderful right out of the oven, or frozen and reheated whenever they are needed.

Servings: 12

Ingredients:

1 cup quick cooking oats
1 cup buttermilk
1 cup flour
1 teaspoon salt
1 teaspoon baking soda
1 egg
1/2 cup brown sugar
1/2 cup vegetable oil

Method:

Soak oats in buttermilk for 2 hours.
Preheat oven to 425 degrees.
Sift flour, salt, baking powder, and baking soda.
Add egg, brown sugar, and oil to oatmeal mixture. Carefully add flour mixture.
Bake in greased muffin tins for 25 to 30 minutes.

Each serving contains:

Calories: 193
Protein: 3 grams
Carbohydrates: 22 grams
Fat: 10 grams

Watch 'em Grow Popovers

Children will love watching these grow in the oven. Add fruit spread or just eat them plain. What a great addition to any meal!
Servings: 6

Ingredients:

3 eggs
1 cup milk
3 tablespoons margarine, melted
1 cup flour
1/2 teaspoon salt

Method:

Preheat oven to 375 degrees.
Generously grease six 2-inch deep custard cups.
On low speed, beat eggs until frothy. Add milk and melted margarine. Add flour and salt. Beat until smooth.
Fill custard cups 3/4 full.
After baking 1 hour, slit top of each popover to let out steam. Bake additional 10 minutes.
Remove popovers immediately from cups. Serve hot.

Each serving contains:

Calories: 184
Protein: 7 grams
Carbohydrates: 18 grams
Fat: 9 grams

Cinnamon Cream Cheese Bites

These bite-sized and tasty appetizers or snacks are sure to be a hit, so make a large batch.

Servings: 12

Ingredients:

6 slices soft white bread
1/2 cup soft cream cheese
3 tablespoons sugar
1 teaspoon cinnamon
1/2 teaspoon nutmeg
1/4 cup melted margarine

Method:

Preheat oven to 350 degrees.
Trim crust from bread.
Spread cream cheese evenly among bread slices.
Roll bread into logs. Cut each log in half.
Mix sugar, cinnamon, and nutmeg together in small bowl.
Using pastry brush, coat each with melted margarine. Roll in sugar mixture. Set on cookie sheet.
Bake for 10 to 12 minutes or until lightly browned. Cool slightly.

Each serving contains:

Calories: 119
Protein: 2 grams
Carbohydrates: 10 grams
Fat: 8 grams

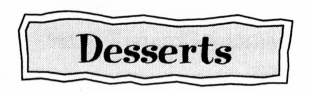

Lemon Zucchini Cookies

No one will ever know there's zucchini in these cookies. It's a great way to incorporate a green vegetable into your child's diet.
Servings: 4 dozen cookies

Ingredients:

3/4 cup margarine, softened
3/4 cup sugar
1 egg
1 teaspoon grated lemon rind
2 cups flour
1 teaspoon baking powder
2 zucchini, peeled and shredded
1 cup powdered sugar
1 1/2 tablespoons lemon juice

Method:

Preheat oven to 350 degrees.
Cream butter and sugar. Add egg, lemon rind, flour, baking powder, and zucchini. Grease cookie sheet. Drop mixture by spoonfuls onto cookie sheet. Bake for 10 minutes. Cool. Combine powdered sugar and lemon juice to make glaze. Drizzle over cookies while slightly warm.

Each serving contains:

Calories: 67
Protein: 1 gram
Carbohydrates: 9 grams
Fat: 3 grams

Spice Squares

Not only are these squares flavorful, but they make your house smell great while they're baking.

Servings: 2 1/2 dozen

Ingredients:

1/4 cup vegetable oil
1 cup sugar
1/4 cup honey
2 cups flour
1 teaspoon cinnamon
1/2 teaspoon nutmeg
1 teaspoon baking soda
1 egg

Topping:

1 cup confectioners' sugar
1 tablespoon water
1 tablespoon vanilla
2 tablespoons melted margarine

Method:

Preheat oven to 350 degrees.
Combine oil, sugar, and honey. Add remaining ingredients.
Blend well.
Turn mixture into 9 x 13-inch pan. Bake 20 minutes.
While baking, combine topping ingredients.
Pour over warm spice squares.

Each serving contains:

Calories: 103
Protein: 1 gram
Carbohydrates: 19 grams
Fat: 3 grams

Low-fat Lemon Squares

Using low-fat cream cheese and no egg yolks in these lemon squares decrease their fat content. You probably won't be able to tell the difference between these and the higher fat ones.

Servings: 20 squares

Ingredients:

Crust:

1 cup sifted flour
1/4 cup confectioners' sugar
1/4 cup low-fat cream cheese
3 tablespoons vegetable oil

Filling:

3 large egg whites
3/4 cup sugar
1 1/2 tablespoons grated lemon rind
2 tablespoons flour
1/2 teaspoon baking powder
1/4 teaspoon salt
1/3 cup lemon juice
confectioners' sugar

Method:

Preheat oven to 350 degrees.
Spray 8-inch square baking pan with non-stick cooking spray.

Crust: In large bowl, stir together flour and   sugar.
Using pastry blender, cut cream cheese into flour mixture until crumbly. Gradually add oil, stirring with a fork. (The mixture will be crumbly.) Press into bottom of prepared pan.
Bake 20 to 25 minutes until light brown.

Filling: In mixing bowl, beat egg whites, sugar, and lemon rind until smooth.
In separate bowl, mix together flour, baking powder, and salt. Add to egg white mixture and blend. Stir in lemon juice.
Pour filling over hot crust.
Bake 20 minutes longer or until top is golden brown and set. Cool.
Dust with confectioners' sugar.

Each serving contains:

Calories: 90
Protein: 2 grams
Carbohydrates: 14 grams
Fat: 3 grams

Oatmeal Raisin Cookies

Keep these in your cookie jar (if you can). They're nutritious, delicious, and everyone loves them.

Servings: 36 cookies

Ingredients:

1 cup flour
1/2 teaspoon baking soda
1/4 teaspoon cinnamon
1/4 teaspoon nutmeg
1/2 cup margarine, softened
2/3 cup light brown sugar
1 egg
1 teaspoon vanilla
1 cup rolled oats
3/4 cup raisins

Method:

Preheat oven to 350 degrees.
Combine flour, baking soda, cinnamon, and nutmeg. Set aside.
In large bowl, cream margarine and brown sugar. Add egg and vanilla. Slowly add flour mixture and blend well.
Stir in oats and raisins.
Drop dough by teaspoonfuls on lightly greased cookie sheets.
Bake 10 to 12 minutes until golden brown.

Each serving contains:

Calories: 70
Protein: 1 gram
Carbohydrates: 10 grams
Fat: 3 grams

Carrot Brownies

Who would even guess there are carrots in these? They'll soon be a family favorite.

Servings: 2 1/2 dozen

Ingredients:

1/2 cup margarine
1 1/2 cups firmly packed
  brown sugar
2 cups flour
2 teaspoons baking powder
1/2 teaspoon salt
2 eggs
2 cups grated carrots

Frosting:

2 ounces (2/3 of 3 ounce
  package) cream cheese
1/3 cup margarine, softened
1 teaspoon vanilla
1 1/2 cups confectioners' sugar

Method:

Preheat oven to 350 degrees.
In large saucepan, melt margarine. Add brown sugar. Stir until blended. Remove from heat.
Combine flour, baking powder, and salt in small bowl. Set aside.
Beat eggs into slightly cooled mixture. Add flour mixture and carrots. Blend well. Pour mixture into 9 x 13-inch pan.
Bake 30 minutes.
Combine frosting ingredients. Frost brownies when cool.

Each serving contains:

Calories: 151
Protein: 2 grams
Carbohydrates: 23 grams
Fat: 6 grams

Bread Pudding

Everyone's favorite. Keep this recipe handy for an easy end-of-a-meal treat.

Servings: 10

Ingredients:

2 cups milk
4 tablespoons margarine, softened
2 eggs
1/3 cup sugar
1/2 teaspoon cinnamon
1/4 teaspoon salt
1 teaspoon vanilla
4 slices soft bread, torn up into chunks
1/2 cup raisins

Method:

Preheat oven to 350 degrees.
Heat milk to boiling and add margarine.
Beat eggs. Add milk and margarine.
Add sugar, cinnamon, salt, and vanilla.
Spread bread chunks and raisins into lightly greased casserole dish.
Pour milk mixture over bread.
Set casserole dish in larger pan filled with 1-inch hot water. Bake 50 to 60 minutes until knife inserted in center comes out clean.
Serve hot or cold.

Each serving contains:

Calories: 157
Protein: 4 grams
Carbohydrates: 20 grams
Fat: 7 grams

Chocolate Peanutty Banana Lollipops

A fun, creative snack or party food. You may have to double the recipe.

Servings: 8

Ingredients:

4 firm bananas
3/4 cup peanuts, finely chopped
3/4 cup chocolate chips
1 tablespoon vegetable oil
8 popsicle sticks

Method:

Cover cookie sheet with waxed paper.
Peel bananas, cut in half, and insert popsicle stick into each.
Heat oil and chips over low heat until melted and mixture is smooth. Remove from heat.
Spread mixture over bananas with spoon. Roll into chopped nuts.
Place on cookie sheet.
Refrigerate until firm, about 20 to 30 minutes.

Each serving contains:

Calories: 227
Protein: 5 grams
Carbohydrates: 25 grams
Fat: 14 grams

Orange Fruit Pie

This colorful, attractive, and light dessert is sure to bring you compliments galore. Let your children help decorate it with fruit.

Servings: 12

Ingredients:

1 cup water
1 3-ounce package orange gelatin
8 ounces sour cream
1 prepared graham cracker pie crust
2 cups fresh fruit, cut up
   (strawberries, grapes, cantaloupe, bananas, kiwi)

Method:

Boil water and dissolve gelatin. Add sour cream.
Chill mixture until slightly thickened, but not set.
Spoon mixture into crust. Chill until set, about 2 to 3 hours.
Top with fresh fruit before serving.

Each serving contains:

Calories: 215
Protein: 8 grams
Carbohydrates: 21 grams
Fat: 11 grams

Rainbow Fruit Kabobs

Here's a great recipe for little helpers. Serve to guests, both older and younger.

Servings: 8

Ingredients:

1/2 cup strawberries
1/2 cup blueberries
1/2 cup green seedless grapes
1/2 cup red seedless grapes
1/4 cantaloupe, cut in cubes or balls
wooden picks/skewers

Method:

Wash fruit. Cut leaves off strawberries.
Cut cantaloupe into balls or cubes.
Carefully spear fruit using various colors on each stick
to resemble a rainbow.
Serve as a snack or dessert.

Each serving contains:

Calories: 26
Protein: 0 grams
Carbohydrates: 6 grams
Fat: 0 grams

Frozen Rainbow Sandwiches

Easy, yet delicious. Make extra—you'll go through these fast.
Servings: 4

Ingredients:

8 graham cracker squares
1/2 cup rainbow sherbet

Method.

Let sherbet thaw at room temperature about 15 minutes.
Spread 2 tablespoons softened sherbet between
2 graham cracker squares.
Wrap each sandwich in plastic wrap. Freeze until firm.

Each serving contains:

Calories: 94
Protein: 1 gram
Carbohydrates: 18 grams
Fat: 2 grams

Orange Yogurt Popsicles

A light, delicious version of an old favorite: dreamsicle. Children love to help make these special treats.

Servings: 8

Ingredients:

1 6-ounce can frozen concentrated orange juice, thawed
1 pint plain low-fat yogurt
2 teaspoons vanilla extract
1/4 cup sugar

Method:

Combine ingredients. Fill popsicle molds.
Freeze until firm, about 24 hours.

Each serving contains:

Calories: 94
Protein: 3 grams
Carbohydrates: 18 grams
Fat: 1 gram

Baked Apple Cobbler

Crispy, delicious, and great for holidays and special meals. Make even more nutritious by sprinkling wheat germ on top.

Servings: 6

Ingredients:

4 cooking apples, peeled and sliced
6 tablespoons water
1/4 cup flour
1/4 cup sugar
1/4 cup margarine, melted
1/4 teaspoon cinnamon
1/4 teaspoon nutmeg

Method:

Preheat oven to 350 degrees.
Place apple slices equally in 4 custard cups.
Sprinkle 1 tablespoon water over each cup.
Combine remaining ingredients and mix together.
Sprinkle over apples.
Bake 20 to 25 minutes until crumb topping is golden brown.

Each serving contains:

Calories: 167
Protein: 1 gram
Carbohydrates: 25 grams
Fat: 8 grams

Apple Cheese Crisp

Desserts can be nutritious. Try this one and you'll admit it's definitely a winner.

Servings: 10

Ingredients:

8 medium apples, pared and sliced
1/2 cup water
1/2 cup brown sugar
1/2 cup sugar
2/3 cup flour
1/4 teaspoon salt
1 teaspoon cinnamon
1/3 cup margarine
1 cup shredded cheddar cheese

Method:

Preheat oven to 350 degrees.
Arrange apple slices in greased 2-quart baking dish. Add water.
Combine sugars, flour, salt, and cinnamon. Cut in margarine with a pastry cutter until mixture is consistency of cornmeal.
Lightly stir in cheese.
Cover apples with sugar mixture. Bake, uncovered, for 1 hour.

Each serving contains:

Calories: 267
Protein: 4 grams
Carbohydrates: 42 grams
Fat: 10 grams

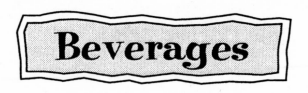

Beverages

Sherbetty Fruit Punch

For a party or just for the fun of it.
Servings: 20

Ingredients:

1 quart orange juice
1 quart pineapple juice
2 cups club soda
1 quart orange sherbet

Method:

Stir together orange juice, pineapple juice, and club soda.
Carefully add sherbet and mix until smooth.

Each serving contains:

Calories: 102
Protein: 1 gram
Carbohydrates: 23 grams
Fat: 1 gram

Yogurt Strawberry Smoothie

Nutritious, delicious, and a great quencher on a warm day.
Works well with other fruit, too.

Servings: 4

Ingredients:

1 pint plain low-fat yogurt
2 cups fresh strawberries
1/4 cup sugar
1/4 teaspoon vanilla extract

Method:

Combine all ingredients in blender.
Blend until smooth.

Each serving contains:

Calories: 143
Protein: 6 grams
Carbohydrates: 26 grams
Fat: 2 grams

Index

underweight children, 62-63
unsaturated fats, 67
utensils, using, 45

vegan diet, 10
Vegetable Dip, 142
Vegetable Pizza Pocket, 135
vegetables, 29, 105, 110, 138-145
vegetarianism, 10, 71
Veggie Chowder, 122
vitamin supplements, 71, 103
vitamins, 6-8, 9
vomiting, 35, 60

Watch 'em Grow Popovers, 156
water, 8, 27
weaning, 27, 36, 45
weight,
    children's, 37, 62-65, 66, 77
    mother's, 2-4, 5
weight gain, pregnancy, 3, 4
weight reduction, 63
wise food choices, 58

Yogurt Strawberry Smoothie, 173
Your Own Baked
    Chicken Nuggets, 126
Yum Yum Salad, 147